CHILD'S NAME _____

Immunization Record

DOCTOR'S NAME _____

		DATE	AGE	REMARKS
Diphtheria	First			
Tetanus	Second			
Whooping Cough	Third			
	Boosters			
Polio	First			
	Second			
	Third			
	Boosters			
TB Test				
Rubella				
Measles				
Mumps				
HIB				
Chicken Pox				

Bring this book to the office. Ask your healthcare provider to enter your child's immunizations as they are administered. This is valuable information to you, and if you should move to another location, for your new clinician. See chapter 12 for further discussion on vaccination schedule and communicable diseases of childhood.

This book does not take the place of your doctor. Different people react differently to the same treatment, test, or procedure. You should always consult your doctor before undertaking any course of treatment.

Neither the author nor the publisher take responsibility for any possible consequences of any course of action suggested in this book. Always call your doctor if you have a question.

Other books in this series which may be of interest:

A Miracle in the Making

Pregnancy

A Doctor Discusses Nutrition
During Pregnancy and Breast Feeding

Breast Feeding

A Doctor Discusses Your Life
After the Baby is Born

A Guide to Pregnancy and Childbirth

a doctor discusses

The Care and Development of

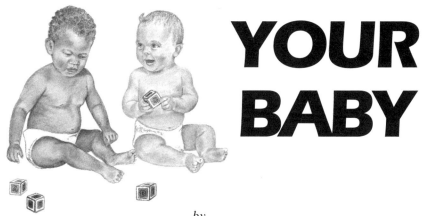

YOUR
BABY

by
MAY GUY M.D. and MIRIAM GILBERT

Illustrated by
LYNN NEMRAVA

BUDLONG PRESS COMPANY • Chicago, Illinois 60631-1032

Table of Contents

CHAPTER 1

Your Baby Is Born

THE ARRIVAL OF A BABY is tremendously exciting - whether it is your firstborn or the addition of a little brother or sister to the family. It can also prove to be pretty baffling if this is your first or you have not been around newborn babies for a long time. Learning something of what to expect of babies at different ages can often help the mother of a new baby cope with problems and situations that are "old". Of course, there is no substitute for experience. Most parents are more relaxed and knowledgeable with subsequent babies than they are with the firstborn. Every baby, however, is different from every other, even in the same family. Almost all of them go through the same stages of development, although at different rates.

The sound of your baby's first cry will be music to your ears. It is also nature's way of proclaiming that the baby is vigorous. And it helps him to fill his lungs with air.

No matter what you may have preferred beforehand, the moment the doctor announces "It's a girl!" or "It's a boy!", your disappointment evaporates. You know that you would never have wanted him or her otherwise.

For easier writing we will assume the baby is a boy. Thus we will not have to say "he or she" each time.

Although you may be tired and groggy, more than likely you are curious to know what happens to your baby immediately after birth. The doctor who delivers the infant quickly checks to see that he is well-formed and that his color is good. The umbilical cord is then cut. There is no sensation in the cord so the cutting is not painful. It was through this narrow "pipeline" that your baby received his nourishment and oxygen. Through it he passed off waste products. About a two inch stump is left on the baby's navel. It is tied off or clamped so that it will not bleed.

The other end of the cord is attached to the placenta or "afterbirth." This, in turn, separates itself from the uterus and is "born." It, too, is carefully checked by the doctor.

WHAT HAPPENS TO BABY AFTER HE IS BORN

Now baby is on his own. His ability to regulate his circulation, temperature and breathing are all carefully watched during the first twenty-four hours by expert nurses and doctors. They make frequent checks of skin color, temperature, heart rate, breathing rate and regularity and general vigor. They also give baby a "grade" on each of these points, according to the APGAR rating. This was devised by Dr. Virginia Apgar in order to keep close track of a baby's vital signs immediately after delivery. This is especially important for premature babies because they are more delicate.

BONDING

Much has been said about the importance of bonding. Researchers have found that early parent-child bonding (from birth to three years) is important for a child's development as well as for parent-child relationships. In addition, there is some evidence that when bonding occurs the family group is strengthened and future child abuse may be decreased.

Early bonding consists of close physical and emotional attachment. Cuddling, kissing, and holding are important in bonding as are eye contact (it has been shown that a baby can often follow the parent's eyes immediately after birth) and breastfeeding.

Generally, the earliest bonding occurs immediately after delivery when the newborn is placed on the mother's stomach. If she is up to it, the mother might want to try breastfeeding. Be aware, however, that this action is primarily emotional. A new mother doesn't usually begin to lactate fully for another two to two-and-a-half days.

If you are not able to take advantage of a birthing room or rooming-in facilities (where bonding is most easily accomplished), you can still establish close contact with your baby in the delivery room, during feeding periods, and later at home.

IDENTIFICATION

Some sort of identification band is placed on the baby while he is still in the delivery room. A footprint or handprint is also taken.

PROTECTIVE CARE AND TESTS

Drops or an ointment are placed in baby's eyes to prevent possible infection. The medication added may be silver nitrate or an antibiotic such as erythromycin.

If the baby shows any signs of early jaundice, such as yellow skin and eye-balls, or if the tests made on the mother indicate a need for it, the baby's blood will be tested for Rh factor and antibodies. In many places, tests are also routinely run to determine potential PKU imbalance, hypothyroidism and protein metabolism problems. If positive (a relatively rare occurrence), these tests are best explained by your doctor.

THE DOCTOR'S EXAMINATION IN THE HOSPITAL

Your baby's doctor, as well as the pediatric resident doctor, will make a thorough examination of the baby in the nursery. He will note the weight, height and circumference of the head. The average full term baby weighs between six and eight pounds, and is about nineteen to twenty-one inches long. Always remember that there is a wide range of normal variation. "Average" means that some babies will weigh more and some less and still be normal. During the first twenty-four hours a baby loses much water from the somewhat waterlogged tissues so the weight may decrease by as much as a quarter to a half pound. After this initial loss of weight which is more apparent than real, it will be several days before the baby starts to gain weight. It may take a week to ten days for him to regain his birth weight. In the meantime, his body is busy adjusting to life in the outer world.

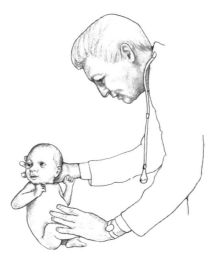

GENERAL APPEARANCE OF THE BABY

A newborn baby lies in a compact little bundle. The head is rather large in proportion to the body. There is little neck. All new babies tend to have a receding chin. This makes it easier for then to nurse. Arms and legs are folded up close to the body almost as in the pre-birth position. Even the feet may be bent inward a little as they were before birth. Notice how tightly baby's fists are clenched. They will remain that way for the next five or six weeks and only gradually open out.

It is comforting to know that your baby's appearance will change and improve from day to day. For example, bruises and skin discoloration generally clear up in short order.

BABY'S COLOR. There may be some temporary blueness on parts of the baby which were pressed on during delivery. This may take a day or so to disappear. Any generalized blueness will be watched by the doctor and nurses. A thorough check will be made of heart and lungs. Oxygen may be required for a time. The amount of oxygen given is carefully monitored, especially in premature babies.

BABY'S SKIN. The skin of a newborn baby looks wrinkled because there is little or no subcutaneous fat to give the rounded appearance which comes later. The skin is very thin, allowing tiny veins to show through. This occasionally gives the baby a mottled appearance. Fairly often there are tiny pink birthmarks, especially on the back of the neck or face. These show up redder when the baby cries or is warm but are temporary and gradually fade. Sometimes there are tiny white spots over the nose called *miliaria*. These disappear.

HAIR AND NAILS. A newborn baby may have a surprising amount of hair. If the baby is on the immature side, hair and nails may be scanty. A fine, downy type of temporary hair, called *lanugo*, may appear on the face.

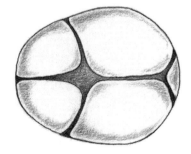

BABY'S HEAD. The head is often out of shape because of the necessary molding as it passes through the birth canal. The skull bones are still soft and have not yet grown together. This allows them to slide over one another during labor. The doctor examining the baby can feel all of these suture lines and particularly the two *fontanelles* or "soft spots" where these suture lines come together. The soft spot near the front is larger. It will not close over for some months. It is covered, however, with tough, durable skin and membranes so that you do not have to be afraid to touch or wash it thoroughly.

If the trip through the birth canal was a little difficult, there may be a lumpy bruise on one side of the head or the neck. This is called a *hematoma*. It is harmless but will take some time to absorb and disappear. All these things your doctor will examine for and explain to you.

BABY'S EYES, EARS, NOSE AND MOUTH. The baby tends to hold his eyes partly shut. He closes them completely when crying. The examining doctor will have to open the eyes gently to check them.

The ears may seem floppy as cartilage has not yet hardened. There are many variations in the shape of the ears.

The doctor will look in the baby's mouth with a flashlight and tongue blade to see that there is no abnormality of the palate, such as a cleft; or of the tongue, as in tongue-tie. The latter causes no trouble and on this score the doctor will reassure you.

BABY'S CHEST. The baby's chest is small and narrow, deeper than wide. Among the first things a doctor listens for with the stethoscope are the baby's breathing and breath sounds, the heart rate and heart sound. These rates are both normally more rapid in a newborn and not so regular as they will be later. Heart murmurs may be heard which may be temporary and disappear, or merit further observation later.

BABY'S ABDOMEN. The baby's abdomen is rather prominent. The cord stump on the navel is a two or three inch bluish-white, soft tube with a tie or clamp on the end. The doctor will inspect it to be sure it is clean, dry and not oozing.

BREAST AND GENITALIA. Occasionally the breasts in a newborn boy or girl will be somewhat swollen and appear to be secreting a little milk from the nipples. This is an endocrine effect from the mother. It is temporary. The doctor will advise you, if it should occur in your baby, that it is of little significance. There is one important precaution, however. *Under no circumstances should any attempt be made to squeeze the secretion from the breasts.* They should be left alone except for some gentle bathing.

In girl babies there may be another hormone effect in the form of mucus secretion from the vagina. This is also temporary. The genitalia are prominent in newborns. Hospital nurses will usually show you how to cleanse a girl's genitalia.

5

In examining a boy's genitalia, the doctor gently feels in the scrotum to see if the testicles are fully descended. When testicles are undescended, the scrotum looks small and empty. The penis of a newborn boy has a long adherent foreskin over the tip. This usually cannot be retracted. It is this part which is removed by circumcision.

BABY'S EXTREMITIES (Arms and Legs). The doctor examines these to be sure they are well-formed and move freely. He or she tests their range of motion, particularly checking the hips to rule out congenital dislocation, and checks the feet to see if they show any effects of pressure from the prenatal position. For instance, the feet might be turned in a bit, similar to "pigeon toes." This may straighten itself out in time. An extreme case may require special treatment later. Sometimes the simple maneuver of switching the baby's shoes to the "wrong" feet helps straighten them out. It is wise to consult your doctor before doing this.

BABY'S REACTIONS. Many of these are automatic during the first weeks. A pat on the cheek makes baby turn his head to that side as if he expected food to come from that direction. Anything that touches the lips will cause sucking motions, whether it is food or not. Touch the bottom of a baby's foot and his toes will curl around your fingers.

The most dramatic of these early automatic reactions is the Moro reflex for which the doctor always tests. In response to a sudden jolt or possibly even a loud sound, the baby suddenly flings his arms and legs outward as if startled. Indeed it is sometimes called the "startle reflex." It is similar to the reaction of your knee jerking when a doctor hits it with a rubber reflex hammer. The Moro reflex indicates to the doctor that all the nerve and muscle connections to the baby's arms and legs are intact. At times newborn infants seem "trembly." This is only an early immature reaction that is *temporary*.

DECISIONS

There are several decisions that you and your partner will have to make. Some member of the hospital staff will ask you about them. It is wise to be prepared with your answers ahead of time.

They include the following:

1. Choosing the baby's doctor (unless the doctor who delivers the baby will also care for him).
2. Type of feeding, whether breast or bottle.
3. If a boy, do you want him circumcised?

YOUR BABY IS BORN

BABY'S DOCTOR

If the doctor who delivered your baby specializes in obstetrics, he or she may recommend a baby doctor for you. Or you may rely on the recommendations of your friends. You may prefer general practice family doctors who will give you prenatal, obstetric and also pediatric care for the baby. The baby will be examined in the hospital not only by your baby's doctor but also by the resident hospital physician.

CIRCUMCISION

Circumcision if the practice of removing the foreskin from the penis of baby boys. It is one of the most common surgical procedures performed in the United States.

In 1975, a special report of the Ad Hoc Task Force on Circumcision took the position that there were no valid medical indications for the routine circumcision of the newborn.

However, in the early 1980's, uncircumcised boys were found to be at a higher risk for urinary tract infections during infancy. Other benefits of circumcision in the newborn were noted in subsequent studies. These benefits include helping prevent sexually transmitted diseases, lowering the risk of problems affecting the penis (including possibly cancer), new evidence that circumcision may offer some protection against the human immunodeficiency virus (HIV) infection, the virus that causes AIDS. The risks of complications from circumcision of newborn baby boys is extremely low.

As a result of the new findings, the American Academy of Pediatrics Task Force on Circumcision, released a report in 1989 significantly different from their original report. The new report now states there are "potential medical benefits and advantages" of newborn circumcision. Since this new report was issued, a number of physicians - even some who participated in efforts to originally reduce the frequency of circumcision have altered their position and now endorse routine circumcision in newborn baby boys.

Information collected in four studies, and reported in the Feb 1992 edition of the Journal American Medical Association, has demonstrated a higher incidence of urinary tract infections in infants who have not been circumcised. It appears likely that the foreskin provides a moist surface that promotes growth of bacteria into the space between the intact foreskin and the glans.

Some parents want their sons circumcised for religious reasons. At one time this was done before the baby left the hospital. Now because of the brief hospital stay after birth, the procedure is usually done either in an out patient facility or at home. The penis heals in a few days and very rarely are there any complications.

Customs are slow to change. If you feel you want to have your son circumcised but are confused by the new guidelines, discuss it with your doctor. Do this during one of your prenatal visits so you have plenty of time to make an educated decision. Your doctor can answer your questions and help you to choose what is best for your child.

BREAST OR BOTTLE

In these early months, the major portion of baby's waking moments are connected with feeding. For this and many other reasons, the decision you make on breast vs. bottle feeding (or a combination of the two) is one of the most important. Rest assured, however, that, whatever you decide, your newborn will thrive as long as you follow a few simple guidelines.

The American Association of Pediatrics strongly encourages breastfeeding. There are so may benefits to both baby and mother that breastfeeding should be the only feeding for baby during his first six months. For a more detailed discussion of breastfeeding vs formula feeding, see Chapter 3. Cow's milk should never be given to baby before the age of one year.

Chapter 2

Baby Comes Home

YOU HAVE JUST COME HOME WITH YOUR NEW BABY. Before we discuss what you can expect from your baby, it is important to be aware of the major health problems that can occur from environmental tobacco smoke or ETS.

Researchers have found that breathing someone else's smoke is very dangerous, especially for children. ETS is defined as the smoke breathed out by a smoker and includes the smoke that comes from the tip of a burning cigarette. ETS has almost 4,000 chemicals in it that infants and children breathe in whenever someone smokes around them, according to the American Academy of Pediatrics. Children who inhale ETS are at risk for many serious health problems including upper respiratory infections, ear infections, and asthma, as well as causing problems for children later in life.

Therefore, if you smoke - quit. If you must smoke, do not do it in your home. It is important not to allow anyone else to smoke in your home. Do not take your baby to any facility where he/she will be exposed to ETS.

Do not be afraid to handle your baby, just be sure to support his head and back when you lift him. He will not be able to hold his head up without support for several months. There is a useful baby appliance, the infant seat,

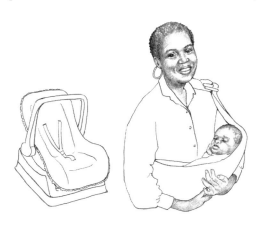

which supports head and back well. He can be propped up in it a little as a change from his crib. It makes a good carrier, too, when baby is ready to be taken out. Do **not** use it, however, for your car. Infant car carriers are specially designed for this purpose. (See Chapter 17). For closer human contact when you're walking, you may want to buy the many varieties of front - and backpacks which are on the market.

It is helpful to know what to expect of your baby so that you won't expect too much too soon. Each baby establishes his own pace and pattern of development. Yet many similarities exist among babies at particular stages of growth. In general, girl babies develop faster than boys. This does not mean they end up any brighter or better. Some babies will do things earlier and some later and still be within the normal range.

DOES BABY SEE YOU? CAN HE HEAR MUCH?

Extensive research on newborn awareness has shown that although babies do not realize they exist in the same way we do, their range of perceptions from the first moment is truly astonishing. Ten minutes after birth, a baby can localize sound. He prefers patterns over solids and stripes and angles over circles. He reacts to unpleasant odors and after the third or fourth day, distinguishes between sweet and bitter tastes. In short, he is not merely a passive receiver; he is ready to react to the world.

Admittedly, a newborn is still greatly limited, a factor which sometimes results in frustrated crying. His ability to focus, for instance, is restricted to about seven to eight inches. Do not be concerned if you notice occasional crossing of the eyes. This is part of the eye muscle-nerve development in the early months.

You will soon find that the newborn responds to tones and volumes of voice, footsteps, and even soft music or the whir of an engine. In general, you should not have to keep your household unusually quiet for him to sleep. Neither can baby be expected to sleep through a blasting radio or TV program. Sudden loud noises or jerky handling may cause the "startle" reflex mentioned previously. This does not mean, as some mistakenly think,. that the baby is "nervous."

BABY'S ACTIONS AND RESPONSES

A new baby's reactions to touch and jarring are rather automatic. His other motions are seemingly aimless waving of arms and legs, and shallow, sometimes irregular breathing. As the voluntary control of the baby develops, the early automatic responses drop out.

The newborn does not have very sophisticated equipment for responsiveness as yet but you will somehow sense that he likes to be held and cuddled and that he enjoys the sound of your voice. The same faces coming repeatedly into his view will provide him with a reassuring human pattern. These are the intangibles that give you the "feel" of your baby and help to prevent some unnecessary crying. A little later he will snuggle into your arms as if he enjoyed it.

WHAT TO EXPECT OF BABY'S DEVELOPMENT

The order of every baby's development is the same. It begins at the head and progresses downward. The eyes come under control first, then the head is held up. Next the arms reach out and finally the back "stiffens" so he can sit. Lastly, the legs support him and, glory of glories, he can walk! All this happens during the first year or so, at different times for different babies but always in this order.

It is important to understand how your baby grows because you will then know what to do for him. It is also of help in choosing and knowing when to use the best appliances for him. There often are spurts of growth alternating with periods of apparently no outward development. Do not push or pressure baby into doing things too soon. Take pleasure and pride in your baby as he is. Enjoy and support his new abilities as he grows.

EARLY ROUTINES

The business of taking care of a baby should be handled in an efficient manner. That way you won't be overwhelmed with tasks. The first few days at home may be hectic. But you are the boss. You should be able to arrange some semblance of organization in the many routines that have to be followed day after day. First, let's consider how the baby is to be dressed.

DRESSING

This should be simple - shirt, diaper, long gown or garment with feet. Socks and booties just do not stay on those squirming feet.

In the early weeks, a cotton blanket folded diagonally around baby's body will not be too confining if you fold it loosely.

Restaining garments with zippers or harnesses should never be used. Also, avoid ribbons or fluffy decorative balls or ornamentation on any garments. They get into baby's mouth too easily.

The lint on new unwashed baby clothes and blankets may tickle your baby's nose and make him sneeze a few times when you dress and undress him. Thus, it might be wise to wash all new clothing once or twice before use.

Despite any covering, a baby's and feet are likely to feel cool to your touch though probably not to him. Room temperature can be kept at whatever is comfortable for you, both night and day.

DIAPERS are baby's best friends. You will need several dozen, depending on whether you use some for pads and towels. The regular diapers are the cheapest. With modern washers and dryers they can be washed daily and kept clean, white and fresh smelling. Modern detergents prevent the gray ammonia-smelling diapers of yore. But stronger detergent powders can leave a residue in the diapers that may cause chemical irritation of baby's skin. It is advisable to use the milder detergents and run the diapers through an extra cycle of the washer for thorough rinsing.

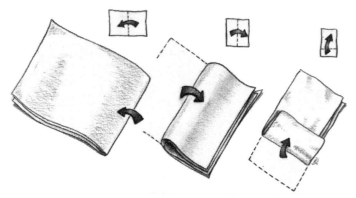

Disposable diapers may be used on trips away from home or at all times if your budget allows it. Although they are difficult to find, diaper liners can be used at times of expected bowel movements. Waterproof pants, which are another convenience, may be hard on baby's skin because they retain warm moisture and keep out air. Many mothers put waterproof pants on babies at night. Some babies cannot tolerate them.

Diapers can be folded either rectangularly or triangularly. For boys, diapers should always have an extra fold in the front; and extra thickness in back is needed for girls.

If you can afford it, a diaper service could be a sanity-saving investment. Generally, these companies wash, boil and deliver enough diapers for your needs, but you should keep a dozen disposables on hand, anyway. If diaper rash should develop, the best treatment is exposure to the air. Leave diapers off at intervals during the day and omit plastic pants at night. Substitute several layers of diapers under the baby instead. If the rash persists, ask your doctor to recommend a good ointment.

Recently, mothers have been encouraged to return to the use of cloth diapers. Not only are cloth diapers recyclable, they are cheaper and better for your baby. It is estimated that a good 16 percent of the contents of a garbage truck are dirty disposable diapers. An estimated 5 million tons of theses diapers are buried annually in landfills, and approximately a third of all disposable diapers contain fecal matter. The feces of infants is known to harbor any of more than 100 viruses including the residues for polio and hepatitis vaccines. Studies have also shown that cloth diapers cause less diaper rashes and infections.

CRIB OR BASSINET?

There is no need to go to unnecessary expense in buying elegant or over-sized baby furniture. What should you get to put baby in at the beginning?

A movable bassinet is a good idea for newborns. It can be easily made by placing a firm pad in an inexpensive plastic clothes basket. You can move the baby from room to room in it. You can place it out of the reach and coughing range of small brothers and sisters who might have colds. Use no pillows nor plastic in or around baby at any time.

At some point, you may want to substitute a crib for the bassinet. If so select one carefully. After 1974, the U.S. Consumer Product safety Commission imposed stringent safety regulations on the manufacture of cribs, but, before then, they were probably the most hazardous item intended for baby use.

Slats should be no more than two and three-eighths inches apart. All metal parts must be smooth-edged. The drop-side railing must be baby proof and securely locked when in the up position, and no side can have railing which could allow baby to climb out when he is older. Finally, the mattress and crib must both be standard size to eliminate spaces where the baby could be pinned in.

If there is any cracked or peeling paint on baby's crib or anywhere in your home, call the health department. Ask them how you can have your home tested for lead paint.

Parents are advised not to place sleeping babies on top of fluffy bedding.

A study by the Consumer Product Safety Commission found up to 30% of 6,000 babies who died of sudden infant death syndrome, had been sleeping on top of soft materials such as comforters and pillows.

A WORD OF WARNING REGARDING WATERBEDS:

In a recent letter to the New England Journal of Medicine, Dr. Enid Gilbert Barnes, professor of pathology from the University of Wisconsin Medical School, reported babies, placed on adult waterbeds, "may be in danger of suffocation or head injuries."

According to Dr. Gilbert Barnes, "Unlike an adult, a baby's small concentrated weight on a large soft area is able to "sink" or form a hole, not allowing it (baby) to move." She also noted a baby was thrown from a waterbed when a sibling jumped up onto the bed.

SLEEPING POSITION

Pediatricians (baby doctors) agree that babies should be placed on their sides or back for sleeping. The American Academy of Pediatrics issued a recommendation in June 1992, that healthy infants be placed on their sides or backs when being put down to sleep and NOT on their stomachs. Babies sleeping on their stomachs are at increased risk for "Sudden Infant Death Syndrome" (SIDS). There may be certain medical conditions affecting some infants where your baby's doctor may recommend your baby sleep on its abdomen. Do not place baby on its abdomen to sleep unless specifically advised to do so by your doctor.

SLEEPING INTERVALS

A new baby may average from ten to twelve sleeping periods a day. Don't expect your baby to do nothing but eat and sleep. Crying periods are to be expected too. Sleeping through the night without waking for night feedings may come at about six weeks or later.

A baby's sleeping periods may vary so much that they upset any attempt you may make towards establishing a regular routine. Don't become over-anxious and feel that it is necessary for baby to get a certain number of hours sleep each day.

CARE OF THE CORD

The cord should be kept as dry as possible. The area around the cord and circumcision can be cleaned but keep the cord itself as well as the circumcision dry. Some doctors suggest an ointment or Vaseline be used on the diaper to prevent the diaper from sticking to baby. It is not necessary to cover these areas with a dressing.

Your doctor may suggest cleaning around the base of the cord with a cotton tipped applicator dipped in alcohol. The cord drops off in about seven to ten days. Then the area may be sponged out with a little alcohol on cotton and a real dunking bath given. Occasionally, there may be a slight crusting discharge in the navel for a few days. If the discharge is very profuse or persistent, it may indicate that a tiny bit of the cord tissue remains. This may require some touching up by the doctor. Once healed, the navel is covered with good, sound skin and you need not be timid about washing it thoroughly.

Hernia of the navel is shown by an outpouching. This is more noticeable when baby cries. Most of these reduce in size as the baby grows and do no harm. Do not tape the navel unless so advised by your doctor.

BATHING A NEW BABY

Bath time can be any convenient time of day. Father might even like to help with it in the evening. Most babies enjoy the bath if the temperature is right and they are held securely.

The only supplies needed are an inexpensive plastic dishpan, one very large towel and some smaller, soft towels and washcloths. Plain soap, not necessarily a baby type, is used. Baby oil and baby powder are not needed. Corn starch, poured first onto the hand and then onto the baby, does just as well. It may be nice to use some lotion in the diaper area when changing baby, but it may be any inexpensive kind, not a special baby type.

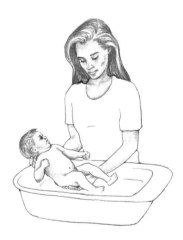

Baby baths are simpler than they used to be. We no longer feel it necessary to poke at or cleanse with Q-tips baby's eyes, ears, nose or mouth. Babies do not need this type of cleansing any more than do adults.

BABY COMES HOME

At first, baby has a sponge bath rather than a "dunking" one because the cord area needs to be kept dry and the circumcision scar, if there is one, will not be healed. You can place a big towel on the counter of the kitchen sink for the sponge bath. Store-bought bathinettes are too tippy and narrow. Include the baby's face, but not the eyes in the soaping process.

"Skate" gingerly around the cord and the circumcision. The normal baby scalp does not have to be bathed more than twice a week.

The genital area of a girl baby is a bit complicated to clean. Use a cloth, cleansing from front to back so as not to go over the rectal area. Cleansing from back to front may transfer harmful bacteria or fungi from the rectal area to the vaginal area, thus causing troublesome irritations and infections. Clean each cleft to the side of the mid-line with a soapy cloth. Remove soap after the cloth is dipped in plain water. Dry gently with a corner of a towel.

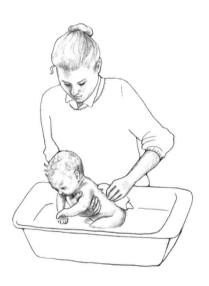

After the cord has come off and the circumcision of a boy has healed, the baby can have a dunking bath. The plastic tub can be placed in the kitchen sink or bath tub with a washcloth or small terry towel on the bottom. Put only a few inches of water in the tub, testing for proper temperature with your elbow. Make sure that the hot spiggot is not directly over the baby and cannot be turned on.

Arrange everything you will need ahead of time - soap, washcloth, towels within easy reach so you will not have to stretch for them after baby is in the tub. Since the baby's head and back need support, hold your hand under his head and upper back when he is in the tub. When washing his back, be sure to support his chest with your arm and to grab his armpit with your hand.

Most mothers find it simpler to soap baby and to cleanse a girl's genitalia before dunking, but others find it easier to soap and rinse one part at a time so baby is not slippery.

BABY COMES HOME

After the baby's bath, pat him thoroughly dry. Pay special attention to drying the creases and folds of armpits and groin. You could put some cornstarch in a talcum powder can to dust in these areas.

Never leave a baby of any age alone in a tub or untended on a high place such as the drainboard or bathinette. NEVER means not even for an instant. If you must answer the phone or doorbell, wrap baby up and take him with you. In this way you will prevent an all to common type of accident.

SUDDEN INFANT DEATH SYNDROME (SIDS)

This section is not meant to unduly frighten you. Rather, it is to make you aware of a condition which you may have read about in the newspapers or in popular magazines.

According to a March 8, 1995 article in the Journal of the American Medical Association, smoking in the same room as an infant, increases the risk for sudden infant death syndrome (SIDS). The more cigarettes an infant is exposed to, the greater the SIDS risk. Passive smoke effects were worse when fathers smoked in the same room as the infant. Breastfeeding helps protect against SIDS among non-smokers, but **not** smokers.

Sudden infant death syndrome occurs without warning and affects approximately two of every 1000 live births. Pediatricians now recommend baby be put to sleep on his back or side and <u>NOT</u> on his stomach (see page 14); this sleeping position helps reduce the risk of SIDS.

The incidence of SIDS varies with different ethnic groups. Asians are at lowest risk; poor African Americans at the highest risk. Two to three months of age seems to be the most vulnerable age and SIDS is rarely seen in infants over six months of age. Boys seem to be at higher risk and in particular, boys who had an earlier infection.

It is also known that infants born of mothers who smoked and/or have a narcotic addiction have a significantly higher risk of SIDS.

What seems to be a common factor among victims of SIDS is the cessation or stopping of breathing during sleep - if this stoppage lasts more than 15 seconds, it is known as apnea, however this association between apnea and SIDS is still controversial.

Infants who would be considered at high risk for SIDS include those who:

1. Have a history of apnea as defined above.

2. A sister or brother who was a victim of SIDS.

3. Have a history of problems related to the pulmonary (lungs), cardiac (heart) and neurological (nerve) systems.

If you believe your infant may fall into this "high risk" category, discuss this and the use of home monitoring devices with your doctor. Though these devices are not 100% effective they may be indicated; your doctor would be the best judge of this.

CAUTION: When taking your baby out for a walk, always carry infant sunscreen with you. Baby has very sensitive skin which must be protected when outdoors.

PETS

A word about pets and your newborn baby. A pet, already an established member within a family prior to the arrival of a newborn, can get jealous if too much attention is paid to an infant.

The American Academy of Pediatrics, in their June 1995 New Release, offers the following advice to pet owners:

- Let your pet and your baby become acquainted slowly.

- Since animals have a keen sense of smell, let your pet sniff the baby's blanket or clothes before you bring baby home.

- Give your pet plenty of attention, also continue to follow your regular play and exercise routine with your pet.

- Never leave a baby alone with an animal - stay no more than an arms length away.

- Make your child's face and hands off-limits to dog or cat kisses. Be alert for symptoms such as wheezing, skin rash and itchy eyes which may indicate an allergy to the animal.

CHAPTER 3

Feeding Your Baby

THROUGHOUT THE 1940's AND 1950's, very few women in the United States breast fed their infants. Even many members of the medical profession seemed to feel that formula was a superior form of nutrition for babies. Starting with the 1960's, more and more research began to demonstrate clearly that human milk is uniquely designed by nature to give the infant nutrients and immunities which bottled milk cannot give.

The advantages to the infant are numerous and significant. Mother's milk is more easily digested and absorbed than formula. It is low in unnecessary minerals to suit the human body's growth rate. It contains rich amounts of protective factors such as immunoglobulins and antibodies to help baby resist diseases, particularly intestinal upsets, and it is virtually free of allergy-producing materials. Breast-fed babies tend less to become obese later in life. The warmth of human contact with the mother encourages psychological attachment.

In addition, there are certain benefits for the mother as well. Breastfeeding is convenient (always ready, at serving temperature, and virtually free from bacterial contamination), it is economical, promotes maternal weight loss, and helps the uterus return to its pre-pregnancy size more quickly. Also, the emotional bonding works for the mother, too, creating ties that can last a lifetime.

However, there may be a valid reason not to breast feed. Probably the most important one is a lack of desire to do so. If you begin breastfeeding only because someone else wants you to, chances are you will not be successful in overcoming the various frustrations you may encounter during the first two or three weeks. Virtually all women who want to breast feed are able to do so.

After discussing the issue with the father and your doctor, make your decision and be comfortable with it. Remember, although you can try breastfeeding and stop if it does not work out, it is much more difficult to change from bottle feeding to breastfeeding and sometimes it can't be done at all.

HUMAN IMMUNODEFICIENCY VIRUS (HIV)

Studies have been reported indicating mothers can transmit the human immunodeficiency virus (the virus that can cause AIDS) to their infants by breastfeeding.

YOUR BREASTS: NURSING, NOT NURSING

There is a mystifying tie-in between the actions of the uterus and the breasts, like two gears meshing. When one works, the other moves. Within three days after delivery, regardless of whether the baby has been premature or on time, some still unknown internal signal sets off the milk-producing mechanism. True, some fluid has been secreted earlier, but this was colostrum, the forerunner of milk.

You will know when the milk is there; the breasts become hard, heavy, full and uncomfortable. For the nursing mother, the soreness will be relieved when the baby begins to suck. The non-nursing mother may have some discomfort during a "drying up" period. Never drink hot liquids while holding baby.

THE NURSING MOTHER

Both you and your baby will require some help and education. In the hospital, a nurse will show you how to place the baby at your breast and techniques for keeping him awake and interested. Generally, the nursing baby will be put to the breast a few times before the milk flows, learning to suck and developing an appetite. But don't let the baby over-nurse at first or your nipples will become sore. The trick is to condition your nipples to the sucking action by letting the baby nurse a few minutes on each breast at each feeding. The colostrum the baby does receive is believed to provide a valuable substance for immunizing him to disease.

It is especially important not to smoke or drink alcoholic beverages if you are going to breast feed. Alcohol is known to pass into breast milk and will closely parallel the mother's blood alcohol level. A baby's liver is very immature and poorly equipped to detoxify alcohol.

TECHNIQUE OF NURSING

When you begin to nurse simply hold the breast against the baby's cheek and he will nuzzle until finding the nipple. A baby instinctively turns the face toward the side that is touched. Hold the breast away from baby's nose so he can breathe easily. Be sure the baby gets a good hold; the mouth should cover the areola, the dark area encircling the nipple. If only the nipple is in the mouth, the baby won't get much milk and will irritate the nipple.

When the baby has finished, do not pull the nipple from the mouth. You have to break the suction gently by placing your thumb on the breast near the baby's mouth and allowing a little air to come between lips and nipple. It's like opening a sealed jar. When you let the air in, it opens easily.

FEEDING YOUR BABY

A nursing mother's nipples do require some extra, tender care. They must be kept clean. Before nursing wash them with water. Rinse well. Sterile gauze pads should be kept over the nipples between feedings.

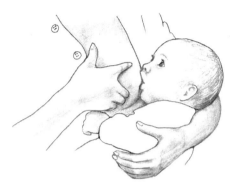

It is not unusual for the nipples to be sore during the first few days of breastfeeding. Do not be alarmed. When lactation is established and the let-down reflex has occurred, mothers frequently describe an increase in fluid pressure which is relieved by the infant sucking. As a rule, the nipples naturally adapt to the nursing experience. If nipple pain continues you should notify your doctor.

In a study of nipple pain it was found that *how* the breast was presented to the baby was the single most important factor. Poor positioning of the baby for breastfeeding during the first few days was the most common cause of painful nipples. Sore nipples are temporary. The breast will gradually adapt to the suckling. The breasts should be exposed to the air as much as possible. Dry heat between feedings may help. Better yet, use an electric hair dryer set on *warm* 6-8 inches away, and fanned across the breast. Many patients bring hair dryers to the hospital with them. After nursing, the breast will be moist. Do *not* wipe dry but allow it to air dry. In some countries, human milk is used to treat skin irritations.

The routine use of ointments to the nipple, areola or breast is not recommended. Lanolin can be particularly dangerous to anyone allergic to wool. Many creams and ointments contain chemicals which may be irritants. Creams with Vitamin E are not recommended unless prescribed by your doctor for a specific problem.

Special nursing bras help support the breasts now heavy with milk. Breasts really have no "muscles" to help them snap back into shape. They are composed of inelastic ligamentous tissues which are best kept from over-stretching by proper bra support. Lack of support can cause breasts to become sagging and pendulous. These practical bras are designed with a handy trap door flap.

The quality of milk produced by the breasts is usually the same sweet rich substance. But it can be affected by extraneous factors. Excitement, anxiety, or deep depression will be reflected in the milk's quality. Drugs, cathartics, alcohol, and nicotine are carried into the milk. These should be eliminated if possible or kept to a minimum. Your hospital diet will automatically include more liquids - you may be treated to a mid-day milk shake.

In the hospital, your baby will be brought to you approximately every four hours depending upon their schedule. If you have a rooming-in plan, you can feed "on demand." You nurse the baby at each breast for about three to five minutes at first, then increase each feeding to ten minutes, then longer when you get home. The more the breasts are nursed, the more milk they will pro-duce. The older and larger a baby grows, the more milk he or she requires and the breasts accommodate to these requirements automatically. When you are home, you may wish to alternate breasts at each feeding. Your doctor will put you on a schedule and decide what is best for your baby's particular needs and your comfort.

Recent studies have reported that healthy, breast-fed babies gain weight at a slower pace than do bottle-fed babies, and suggest that the national stan-dards for normal growth of babies be revised. The present national standards are based on older data when a much higher percentage of women bottle-fed their babies.

How long should you expect to nurse? Pediatricians suggest one year if possible though some babies nurse even longer. However, even six weeks will give your baby an excellent start in life. Two months are even better. Weaning depends upon your baby and you; your doctor can offer practical suggestions.

PROBLEMS THAT MAY ARISE WITH BREASTFEEDING

If baby has a bowel movement at every nursing, do not be concerned. The stools of a breast-fed baby are much looser and unformed than those of a bot-tle-fed baby.

Feeding intervals may be quite irregular at first. A new baby often seems to want to eat every two or three hours and then sleep for a long time. If the long sleep tends to occur during the day, you will have to try to awaken and nurse him every four or five hours. If the long sleeping periods occur at night, let baby sleep. Do the same yourself.

If you have a cold, hand washing is even more important before feeding and handling the baby. You may also drape something loosely over your face, such as a clean dishtowel, to deflect your breath and possible cough away from baby.

An occasional bottle may be given if you wish to get away for a few hours or so to see if baby wants more than he is getting from the breast. This may be simply one ounce of evaporated or two ounces of water (sugar is not necessary), or one of the simple, prepared formulas to which you only add water. You will not want to skip many nursings for it is the regular emptying of the breast by the baby that makes more breast milk come in.

Another alternative is to hand express your breast milk into a sterile bottle. Your doctor or nurse may recommend manual expression - or hand milking of a breast.

MANUAL EXPRESSION

Step 1: After washing your hands, gently and firmly grasp the breast with the thumb above and the fingers under the surface of the breast. Thumb and fingers should rest just outside the areola.

Step 2: Press downward with the thumb on the top of the breast against the fingers cupping the back of the breast. Carry both thumb and fingers downward to the base of the nipple.

Step 3: Pull forward slightly and gently at the back of the nipple - this will cause colostrum to flow during pregnancy or the milk to flow after the baby is born.

EXERCISE

Though moderate exercise is usually not contraindicated during lactation, there have been some studies suggesting that women who exercise excessively, particularly women who jog, may have a problem maintaining an ample milk supply. This may be due to any activity which results in persistent motion of the breasts and excessive friction of clothing against the nipples, and may affect the milk supply. The wearing of a sports or athletic bra made of cotton will reduce this effect.

Studies have also shown elevated levels of lactic acid in breast milk following 30 minutes of aerobic activity (jogging, running, swimming, biking and aerobics). Mothers have reported their infants may reject their milk after strenuous exercise.

Breast milk is very sweet, lactic acid is known to have a sour or bitter taste. Exercise is also known to generate an increase in the amount of sodium and chloride excreted in sweat.

Additional studies are currently ongoing. In the meantime, several precautions are recommended for women following strenuous exercise prior to breastfeeding.

- Shower or at least wash the breasts.

- Manually express and discard 3 to 5 milliliters of milk from each breast.

- If baby puckers his face when given the breast, postpone feeding or replace feeding with previously pumped milked.

TIPS TO THE MOTHER WHO IS BREASTFEEDING

1. Stay on the good diet that you had before baby came. In fact, you should probably step up your caloric level considerably unless you need to lose a great deal of weight.

2. Get plenty of rest. Limit the number of visitors for baby's sake as well as your own.

3. If there is a strong history of allergy in your family, go easy on chocolate, nuts, oranges and other citrus fruits, spices and strongly flavored vegetables. If eggs are used, they should be cooked and never eaten raw, as in eggnog.

4. Once again, *do not take any drugs or medications without your doctor's specific instructions.*

5. For more information on breastfeeding, consult *"Breastfeeding".**

AVOID LOW FAT DIETS

Diets, limiting the fat and cholesterol content for children aged 2 or under, could be dangerous. Skimming the fat and therefore calories from a baby's diet could stunt baby's growth. Cholesterol is necessary to form body cells including those of the central nervous system. By severely limiting baby's cholesterol intake, you could deprive him/her of the cholesterol needed to form these body cells.

Well meaning parents concerned with their baby's becoming overweight, were known to have watered down the infants' formula - some even cut back on fat at meals, used skim or low fat milk, lean meat and eliminated egg yolks.

Doctors at a New York hospital saw first hand, the damage such a diet could cause. Over the past couple of years several children on this type of diet were admitted to a New York hospital with severe growth problems.

FINDING THE RIGHT FORMULA

If you decide to bottle feed, ask your doctor which formula is best. The American Academy of Pediatrics recommends infants under the age of 12 months NOT be given whole cow's milk or low-iron formula.

Finding the right formula may be hard at first, but you have a wide variety on the market to select from. If you want to avoid the fuss, buy canned, ready-to-use formula, but be prepared to pay more. Otherwise, powders or liquid concentrates can be easily diluted with water.

Generally, formulas can have three different bases: cow's milk, soy beans or curd. Goats' milk and meat-based formulas are available but probably hard to find. Almost all babies do fine with the more popular types of formulas, but some infants require a special diet or supplemental nutrients. Also, be prepared to experiment a bit. Babies do have likes and dislikes and digest some foods better than others.

PREPARATION

Follow the directions carefully. Too much or too little water, if you are feeding him formula or evaporated milk, can have a serious cumulative effect. Do not reuse already opened instant formula if it has not been refrigerated. Make sure that the water source is clean and you have proper refrigeration. Clean top of can of formula and all equipment which will be in contact with the formula or with baby. Make sure nipple holes are the right size. If your doctor advises you to sterilize baby's nipples, boil for ten minutes, however, the American Academy of Pediatrics no longer recommends routine sterilization of bottles, formula and nipples.

If your water is from a municipal water supply from a larger city, it is considered safe. If there is any doubt, check with your local water utility. Always use cold water that contains no water softener, for preparing baby's formula.

If you have well water, have your water checked to be sure it does not contain any contaminants. Even trace elements of contaminants, lead, nitrates (from fertilizer), which may not be harmful for adults, are potentially dangerous for young infants. If in doubt about your water supply, use bottled water in baby's formula.

Proper refrigeration of formula is essential. Do not re-refrigerate formula if baby does not finish his bottle.

Feed the bottle within 30 minutes of the time it is made or removed from the refrigerator. If it is not used within an hour, throw out the contents and start with a fresh bottle. Do not refrigerate and re-use a partially consumed bottle.

A word of warning: Many parents will warm infant formula (though it is safe to serve at room temperature). In this age of modern conveniences busy parents warm formula in the microwave oven. There have been reported cases of burns to the roofs of infants' mouths — the bottle felt warm to the touch but the formula itself was too hot. If you feel it is necessary to heat baby's bottle do it on the stove top. If you do use the microwave be certain to test the formula and nipple *before* feeding your infant.

FEEDING POSITION

Hold the baby almost upright when you feed him. Try to sit in a comfortable chair or rocker so you, too, are relaxed. The reason for baby's upright position is to allow for more and better burping. There is always an air bubble in baby's stomach and, as he sucks, he swallows more air. This must be burped up to make room for more milk. If he nurses lying down, the air bubble tends to get under the milk. When the bubble comes, it pushes the milk ahead of it and baby appears to be a "spitter." You can help the bubble to come up by putting baby over your shoulder or leaning him forward on your lap and gently rubbing his back.

For continued spitting up, try slowing down the feeding, burping more frequently during meals, holding him higher, or putting him in an infant seat afterwards to give him a chance to digest. If you are bottle feeding, don't feed baby while he is in an infant seat. The human contact provides an important emotional nourishment. Don't rush him but don't dawdle either. Thirty minutes should be maximum.

FEEDING SCHEDULE

The feeding schedule is likely to be irregular at first. There may not even be any schedule. Baby may want to eat every two or three hours for awhile, then sleep for five or six hours in between. If the frequent wakings are during the day and the less frequent at night, you "have it made." If baby reverses them (and how is he to know the difference between night and day?) try to time it so that he is fed every four hours or so during the day. Remember, though, that an "on demand" schedule is still best.

VITAMIN SUPPLEMENTS

Most doctors now feel that multivitamin supplements, other than A, D and C, are not needed during the non-solid period. The Vitamin B complex and nearly all other minerals are transmitted in full measure through the milk. Nursing mothers in particular, may have to give their babies Vitamin D. In any case, check with your doctor and, more importantly, relax; vitamin and mineral deficiencies are almost unheard of nowadays.

If supplements are called for, ask your doctor about the dosage. It may be mixed with a little of the milk or any liquid, such as fruit juice. Or it may be dropped directly into the baby's mouth, preferably during feeding.

Check to see if your community fluoridates its water. If not, buy a preparation which includes this element, if your doctor so recommends.

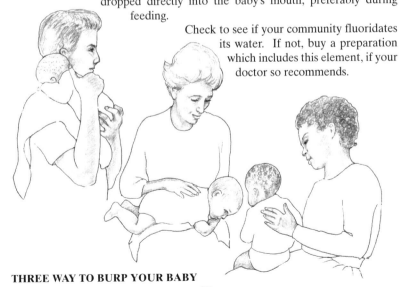

THREE WAY TO BURP YOUR BABY

CHAPTER 4

Crying, A Baby's Communication

THE BABY'S FIRST CRY is a wonderful sound. It lets the mother know that the baby has arrived at last. It tells the doctor that the newborn is vigorous. The deep breaths that accompany the crying are necessary to help expand the baby's lungs. It may take weeks for them to become fully expanded. Crying helps this along, too.

Later, the sound of a baby crying does not sound so pleasing, especially when it seems excessive and the cause difficult to fathom. It may be particularly distressing to a small brother or sister who knows that when he or she cries that hard, there is really something wrong. You will have to explain to them (and perhaps convincing yourself at the same time!) that this is the primary way that the new baby has of communicating his wants and discomforts. It does not always mean that something is seriously wrong.

While you will hear about babies who "do nothing but eat and sleep," they are few and far between. Hardly ever will you hear it said of a firstborn baby. Babies vary a great deal in the amount of crying they do. It can average about two hours a day. Paying attention to baby's crying, and comforting him will *not* "spoil" baby. Comforting and attention are important factors in reinforcing bonds between child and parent.

CAUSES OF CRYING

Most frequently, the baby cries when hungry. You can let baby fuss a little before you rush to feed him, but some doctors believe that a more immediate response on the parents' part results in more patient children. If baby is too sleepy, he is likely to drop off again after the first few mouthfuls have eased the hunger pangs. Sometimes, however, babies, like the rest of us, are simply too tired to fall asleep.

Babies always swallow air when sucking. It is possible that some of the swallowed air goes on through into the intestines and causes a "gas" pain. Such babies tend to pass a good deal of "gas" (really air) by rectum. Extra burping helps relieve these babies and may be necessary for some time after feeding.

Some babies fuss more than others when they are wet or soiled. This cause of crying is easily remedied by more frequent change of diapers. Wetness would be painful to a baby with a severe diaper rash.

Other sources of discomfort for a baby are heat and cold. One is more likely to keep a baby overly warm, especially since his hands and feet normally feel cool to the adult touch. Babies do not perspire very efficiently and may get "heat rash" when bundled up too much.

Some babies have a favorite sleeping position and cry or fuss until placed in this position. More or less you have to go along with this. But try to change the position during waking hours so the baby is not constantly in one position. The bones of a baby's head are still quite pliable at this early age and are likely to show flattening on one side or the back if the sleeping position is not changed. Do not hesitate to pick up your baby fairly often, supporting his back and head with your hand, or to prop him in an infant seat so he won't be in one position all of the time. It is not necessary or desirable to "jiggle" a baby to soothe him.

There is always some crying for which there seems to be no discernible cause. Nothing can be found wrong. It seems as if baby just wants to cry. Such crying occurs more often in the late afternoon or evening as if the baby somehow senses that "things are going on." It may possibly be a bid for some sociability on baby's part. It may quiet him to be out where there are family sounds and light and movement. He can be propped in his infant seat on a firm surface, even on the floor where small brothers and sisters can play around him (if not too rough). Having young children around at this time seems to "register" even with a small baby. Youngsters are down more to his level. Voices are soothing and music that is not too loud will also "register."

Paradoxically, some researchers have found that many babies who cry for no observable reason can be calmed by hearing a tape of themselves crying on another occasion. If you have the equipment, it's worth a try.

TOO MUCH CRYING

When excessive crying continues in the early months without apparent cause, we are prone to call it "colic." The typical colicky baby acts as if he has a tummy ache, doubling up and screaming. Frequent changes of formula and feedings are likely to be tried without much improvement. Some things that might comfort such a baby are: warm water feeding or a pacifier, and a change in baby's position, increasing burping. After three months, as if by magic, this type of crying often disappears.

CRYING, A BABY'S COMMUNICATION

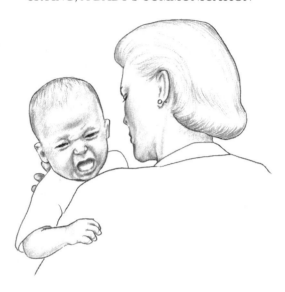

Your doctor may believe that an allergy to cow's milk protein is the reason for your baby's colic. If this is the case, he/she may recommend a hypoallergenic formula called NUTRAMIGEN to help resolve the colic. The protein in Nutramigen is broken down into tiny piece making it easier for baby to digest.

Colic is more frequent in first-borns. Since parents admit that they are more relaxed in their handling of subsequent babies, we have to conclude that parent tension plays some part. Even young babies appear to sense tenseness on the part of the person holding them. This would seem to be an argument against waiting until you are on edge and ready to shriek yourself before picking up your crying baby. You need not fear that a young baby will be "spoiled" by being picked up.

It will be more relaxing to baby if you hold him in a nice comfortable rocking chair and talk or sing to him (the tone of voice gets across) rather than "jiggling" him and walking the floor. Sometimes fathers have a more soothing touch, especially in the middle of the night. This can well be a part of their share in caring for the baby.

SHOULD YOU USE A PACIFIER?

A pacifier is a rubber nipple on a plastic ring. So strong is the sucking reflex in a young baby that he will suck on anything that is placed in his mouth. This naturally diverts him from crying because he cannot suck and cry at the same time, thereby giving a little peace of mind to his parents.

You will find that some people have very strong feelings against using a pacifier and may be heard to say, "I just can't stand to see a baby with a pacifier in his mouth all the time."

Don't let their objections bother you. Often a baby will awaken, cry, and upon being given the breast or bottle, will feed for a minute of two, and go, back to sleep. In such instances, the baby wasn't hungry, he just needed to suck. It's perfectly natural. In fact, sucking gives him training for the day, soon to come, when he will begin to take solid foods. Therefore, you need not feel that you are "playing tricks" on the baby by giving him something to suck on that has no food on the end of it.

One parent, believe it or not, was using the pacifier as a means of reducing the food intake of the baby, lest he develop an obesity problem like the parents. Babies need a lot of nourishment in this early period of rapid growth. They are not likely to become overweight. It is possible that, if too much of their sucking time is diverted by a pacifier, they may not get enough nutrition. It is better to feed a baby more frequently than to give him the pacifier too often.

Some people object that pacifiers can lead to future teeth and jaw deformities. Because most babies will naturally wean themselves off a pacifier in time, this criticism lacks validity. However, to be on the safe side, you should buy orthodontic pacifiers which are designed to keep pressure off the front teeth.

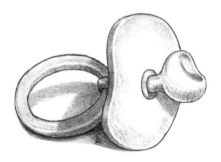

AN ORTHODONTIC PACIFIER

CRYING, A BABY'S COMMUNICATION

If you need one comforting thought to cling to during this difficult period, bear in mind that before long baby's crying will give way to cooing and other more pleasant sounds.

Shaking a baby is a serious form of child abuse and most frequently occurs in babies under the age of 6 months. Violently shaking a baby can cause permanent brain damage resulting in mental retardation, paralysis, and severe motor dysfunction.

CHAPTER 5

Your Baby's First Months and Checkup

IT IS BOTH INTERESTING and important for you to know in which ways your baby's development will be the same or may differ from that of other babies.

DEVELOPMENT AT ONE MONTH

A one-month-old baby lies in a typical "prizefighter position." His head is turned to one side. The arm on that side is stretched out. The other arm is bent close to the shoulder. If you turn baby's head to the other side, his arms may reverse their position. This is of developmental significance, as an illustration of reflexes that are temporary and drop out. Baby may tend to sleep in this position for a time.

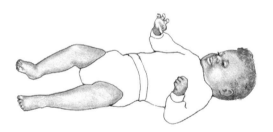

"PRIZEFIGHTER POSITION"

As far as eye development is concerned, baby stares at big things rather vaguely at first and cannot really focus beyond 7 1/2 inches. Gradually, he is able to follow with his eyes a moving object held above him. Such eye development may well be stimulated by occasionally propping the baby in an upright position in an infant seat.

A big moment in his development takes place when baby fixes his gaze on your face and brings forth his first smile. This may appear any time between three weeks and two months. Don't let anyone tell you that it is only a grimace due to "gas" or colic. You will know better for baby definitely smiles and seems to recognize your face.

Another advance occurs when baby begins to lift his head a little when lying prone (on his stomach), although he will quickly drop it again. Do not place healthy baby on his stomach to sleep. He should sleep on his side or back. Most doctors recommend waiting until baby is six months old to add solid foods to his diet. He will be able to lift his head when lying prone before he can do it on his back. You will need to support his head when lifting him for a couple of months yet.

He can now adjust his position somewhat to you, when you pick him up, becoming a little more observably responsive. The types of motion he makes have progressed, too. When on his stomach, he makes crawling motions. When on his back, he thrashes with arms, kicks and pushes with his legs. This makes for fun in the bath. His hands open out from their fisted position and make aimless clutching motions.

SLEEPING

The baby's waking and sleeping periods become more definite than the half drowsing and half rousing periods of the newborn. Gradually he will lie awake for longer periods. Babies vary in this respect, too, some staying awake longer than others without necessarily fussing.

Baby should always be on a fairly firm pad or mattress and never have soft pillows or sheets of plastic, such as plastic bags, around him.

FEEDING

Now the baby can anticipate his feeding. He may stop crying when he sees or hears signs of the bottle or breast. Before he would scream until the nipple was actually placed in his mouth. As he takes more nourishment, baby can wait for a longer feeding interval. He may also sleep through the night. The average number of feedings will then be five or six instead of seven or eight. His schedule will become more regular.

SOLID FOOD. In general, parents are in more of a hurry to start feeding solids than are their doctors. Some allergists feel that feeding solid foods too early might tend to make a baby allergic to some foods. At any rate, nearly all experts agree that now is not the time to start babies on solid foods, contrary to what was thought in the past. An infant should not start with these supplements until he can sit with support and achieves neuromuscular control over his head and neck.

CRYING PERIODS . . .

Crying periods usually decrease after six weeks of age unless you are one of the unfortunate mothers who have to wait out the colicky period. Baby will have several different types of cries. He will also make non-crying sounds like "mew," "coo," and "ah". Feel free to answer back but don't get into the habit of using baby talk. He might just as well hear the correct sounds from the start.

Crying definitely decreases as the baby becomes less preoccupied with his inner sensations and more taken up with the sights, sounds and contacts of the outer world. This is the time to tie rattles and similar toys to the sides of or above his crib. Mobiles are nice, too, hung from the ceiling. You can make one by tying strips of bright paper or cloth on a clothes hanger. Baby will watch these during his wakeful periods.

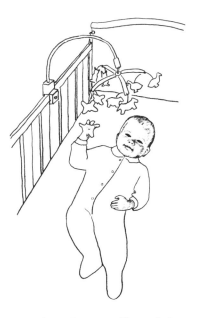

THUMB-SUCKING

Sometime during his second or third month baby may find he has a built-in "toy" at hand. At first, his hand accidentally brushes his mouth, stimulating him to suck it. He quickly learns to put it in his mouth and behold, he has found a handy pacifier that he can drop and pick up at will. Some thumb - or finger - or hand-sucking is part of normal development. It need not be suppressed. It is certainly more sanitary than a pacifier and also gives him the advantage of controlling it himself, sucking when he feels the need.

Considered from a philosophical (and developmental) approach, it is evident that the thumb-sucking baby is going through a normal stage of getting undoubted satisfaction from within himself. If the habit persists into an age when he should be deriving more satisfaction from without, it may be considered undesirable. Many people hate to see an older child sucking his thumb. In most instances, you will find that it is a habit that will disappear as the child grows older and develops outside interests.

SAFETY MEASURES

As you see baby progressing and moving around more, you need to take greater precautions. Never leave a baby of any age alone on a bed without sides or any high place such as a bathinette, even momentarily. He can wiggle an amazing distance at a very young age.

Do not hold a baby of any age while you are having a hot cup of coffee or a cigarette.

Brothers and sisters of toddler age need to be watched lest they put something in baby's mouth, well-meant though it may be.

MEDICAL CHECKUPS

The first medical checkup should occur no later than two weeks of age. This is especially so for the firstborn, mainly because new parents need advice and reassurance. Firstborn do cry more and the new mother or father at least will want some telephone advice on this.

Monthly checkups are usual for the first six months. Baby will be getting monthly immunizations, which start at three months. Later check-ups may be at two, three or four month intervals up to two years of age. minor upsets and special problems usually change any planned interval between checkups. They will also give rise to the numerous telephone calls that a baby doctor gets from parents.

The first year sees the baby almost tripling his birth weight and growing from nine to ten inches, a growth rate so rapid it will never be equalled nor be anywhere near as great in other years.

The minor disturbances for which you are most likely to seek the doctor's help will probably be undue fussiness, skin rashes, spitting up (to differentiate it from actual vomiting), colds and fever. Though most are minor, they can become major. They often seem so to the new parent. Your baby's doctor gives out reassurance more often than prescriptions and will certainly want you to consult him rather than to worry needlessly.

Your doctor will assess your baby's progress at the one month examination and will give you many more pointers than you can read in a book. The following will present some idea of what to expect at the monthly checkup.

THE DOCTOR'S EXAMINATION

Your baby's medical examination at one month is an important occasion. The doctor may have seen the baby for some minor ailment or complaint before this and no doubt there have been some telephone calls from you requesting advice. But this is the first "official" checkup. You should come prepared with a list of questions to ask, things that you may have wondered about. It's well to write your questions down as they arise. Otherwise, when you are in the doctor's busy office, you may forget some of them.

CHECK OF WEIGHT, HEIGHT AND TEMPERATURE

In the office, the usual procedure is as follows:

Baby is completely undressed. All clothing and blankets are removed from wetting distance. A covering diaper should be kept handy, especially for a baby boy, lest you or the doctor or nurse get wet. The baby is then weighed, measured (including head circumference) and has his temperature taken, generally by the office nurse.

Weighing must be done on a good beam scale. Spring scales such as the home bathroom type are never accurate enough. The first month he will average about a pound and a half gain. In the next several months he may increase a good two pounds per month. The height and weight gain vary from one baby to another, especially if they are of different body build.

Measurement of height is not accurate for a wiggling baby unless two people hold him down. But he will probably show an inch of growth as a start toward the eight or ten inches that he achieves by the end of the first year.

It is a good idea for you to watch the nurse when the baby's temperature is taken. Ask for a demonstration of the correct technique so you can take the temperature at home when necessary. The rectal thermometer used should be a broad one and have a broad band of mercury for easier reading. You will be cautioned to wash it under cool water, never hot, The baby is placed on his stomach. The thermometer is lubricated with K-Y jelly or vase-

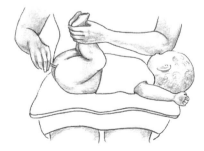 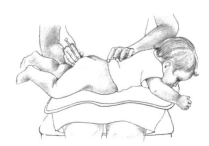

line and inserted into the rectum about and inch. The nurse allows it to take its own direction which is usually slightly downward and forward. It is not necessary or desirable to force it in. With the left hand, the nurse steadies the baby's buttocks and, with the right, holds the thermometer in for a full minute. After withdrawing it and wiping off the lubricant you can see that the "normal" arrow on the thermometer points to 98.6 degrees. This refers to mouth temperature. Rectal temperature is about a degree higher, usually around 99.6 degrees. It is not necessary to transpose it to mouth values when reporting it. Temperature fluctuates normally as much as a degree in the course of a day and night. Anything below 100 degrees is considered normal rectal temperature. You need not be concerned over subnormal readings. They only mean that the thermometer has got into a bit of stool and not against the wall of the rectum. Sometimes the thermometer acts as a suppository, stimulating baby to have bowel movement. Then you have to clean up and start all over again!

Or you may want to buy a battery powered thermometer instead. Although they are not inexpensive, this type of thermometer offers the advantage of giving you baby's temperature almost instantaneously.

WHAT YOUR DOCTOR WILL CHECK FOR

The doctor will note the general appearance of the baby. He or she will examine the baby's skin and scalp, head, neck and chest, abdomen, genitalia, arms and legs, and will check the baby's reflexes.

SKIN AND SCALP. The doctor may note a little scaly "cradle cap" on the scalp, especially over the soft spot. You needn't feel guilty. This growth can develop even if baby's head is carefully kept clean. Applications of vaseline, baby oil, mineral oil, or an ointment the doctor can prescribe will usually make cradle cap vanish.

HEAD AND NECK. The doctor will feel the soft spot, or fontanelle, to see the size. Its width and length will be noted in terms of the doctor's own fingers, that is, one, two, two-and-a-half, or more finger breadths. This way its size and gradual closing can be checked at subsequent examinations. There may be a slight flattening on the back or side of the head remaining from birth or aggravated by a favored sleeping position. The doctor will check the neck muscles to be sure they allow the baby's head to turn equally well to either side.

EYES. You may have noted some crossing of the eyes. The doctor will check this and reassure you if this is part of the normal development. If necessary, he or she will make a note to check it on future visits.

CHEST, HEART AND LUNGS. With the stethoscope the doctor will listen for the heart sound and rate. These are heard better when the baby is not crying whereas the breath sounds in the lungs are better heard when the baby is crying.

ABDOMEN. This is felt by the doctor more easily when it is not tense from baby's crying. The condition of the navel will be noted for hernia or possible discharge.

GENITALIA. If the baby boy has been circumcised, the mark will be checked to see if there are slight adhesions. These the doctor can easily separate at this time. By inspecting the scrotum, the doctor can tell if the testicles are fully descended or can be pushed down readily.

A girl baby may have a tendency to slight filmy adhesions of the vulva (vaginal opening). These are also easily separated. The doctor can show you how to prevent them from forming at home. The deep clefts of the girl's external genitalia are not easy to clean. The doctor or nurse may show you again how to take care of this condition.

EXTREMITIES. The doctor will check to see if the baby's arms and legs move freely and in all directions. He or she will test the range of motion in the hips to rule out any tendency to congenital dislocation.

INFANTILE REFLEXES. The doctor will probably test the baby's Moro (startle) reflex by jerking the pad under him. This reflex begins to drop out in the next few weeks. The tightly fisted hands may also begin to open out now. These are just a few of the ways in which the baby's development is judged.

The doctor's advice on feeding and routines will accompany or follow the examination. Perhaps the most valuable part of this examination and consultation is that it will help to set at rest some of the worries you may have had over the baby. The doctor can also put your mind at ease over superstitions you may have heard. Many false ideas are still held about babies, even by intelligent people. Do not hesitate to ask for the facts.

TELEPHONE CALLS TO THE DOCTOR

New parents handling a baby for the first time need frequent advice. Sometimes all that is necessary is a reassuring word about a minor problem that seems major to them. A baby's doctor expects to get more telephone calls from first-time parents regarding care of the baby in the first month than at almost any other time, except when there is definite illness. At such times the doctor will want you to call and report progress and results of treatment.

To call or not to call is the frequent dilemma of parents who do not want to bother the doctor unnecessarily. It is better to call during the doctor's office hours, if you can, because it gives him or her the chance to look over baby's record and to recall the baby and his history. Very likely the office nurse will take your number, note the complaint and have the doctor call you as soon as possible.

Things have a way of looking worse, whether they are or not, by evening and really bad by the middle of the night. It is better to report to the doctor, if feasible of course, before you get worried. While a doctor will take night calls with good grace, it is most discouraging to hear that the trouble has been going on for two or more days (with ample time to call in the daytime). Yet nobody got really worried until after midnight of the third day. It isn't exactly the best thing for baby, either!

The above is only a suggestion. Never hesitate to call the doctor at any time that a real emergency seems to present itself. More than likely the doctor will make arrangements to see the baby very soon.

PRESCRIPTION FOR EFFECTIVE PHONE CALLS

Here are some other important rules to observe when telephoning your doctor about the baby.

1. Have a pencil and paper by the phone for taking down directions. Have the telephone number of your local pharmacist written down in case a prescription is needed.

2. Make the call yourself. You should give the facts about the baby and not relay them to someone else in response to questions which the doctor may ask.

3. Take the baby's temperature so that you can report it in case of illness. Be sure to give temperature taken by rectum. Do not try to subtract a degree and give it in terms of mouth temperature.

4. Give your doctor your full name and the baby's name and age. Help the doctor identify the baby by reporting the date of the last office visit or offering some other special description.

5. Describe the problem, its duration and symptoms, such as fussiness, undue crying, vomiting, diarrhea, fever, cough, abnormal breath sounds.

6. Learn to be a good observer and accurate reporter. This is the hardest part. It requires experience. Eventually you will realize that the doctor is going to ask certain questions regarding fever, type of cough and breathing, description of rashes, dryness of baby's skin and coloring.

7. While the doctor's telephone advice is a great convenience to you, it is not a substitute for a good office examination and for tests that may be necessary for accurate diagnosis. If the doctor suspects that the baby has something contagious, it may be wise to arrange an office call after office hours.

CHAPTER 6

Your Baby Around Three Months of Age

ONCE YOU GET PAST the first three months, you will be rewarded with a relatively peaceful period. Colicky crying tends to drop out, possibly because baby's intestines are working better instead of "cramping" after food.

The baby's actions are less automatic and gradually come more under control. Previously his hand would automatically close over a rattle that you placed in it. Now his hand does not respond in this automatic way. In time he will develop his own control over his grasp. Probably the first thing he will grasp in this new, more controlled and less automatic manner will be his other hand. It is one of the first things he contacts.

FURTHER SIGNS OF DEVELOPMENT

Your baby is now more of a personality. He smiles at you. He's more "cuddly." He's more aware of his surroundings. He may still jump at loud noises, but it will not be with the same violent fling of the earlier startle reflex. For some time now, he has been able to hold his head up when lying prone. Before you know it, baby will begin to raise himself up on his elbows, too. Suddenly, one day he will roll over onto his back. It will take a little more time before he can raise his head while lying on his back and quite a while longer before he will roll from back to stomach (prone).

Arm control will increase rapidly in the next few months. At first, when you offer baby something, he will become "excited all over." He will wave arms and legs with enthusiasm. When he develops the ability to reach, he does it first with both arms in a jerky sort of way. His next step is reaching with one hand and grasping with all fingers as if he "had a mitten" on his hand. Next he will transfer the rattle from one hand to the other. These are significant advances in control.

FEEDING

Pediatricians and family physicians no longer recommend solid foods at this age. As a rule, solid foods are not added to baby's diet until he is six months old. Breastfeeding or formula preparation should continue.

If you can continue to breast feed your baby that is great! If you feel you have to or want to start weaning baby, you should do so gradually. Begin by substituting one bottle feeding a day for the breast feeding at which you seem to have the least milk. Baby will be familiar with the bottle since he would have had his water from a bottle and possibly some diluted juice. By gradually substituting another bottle for another breastfeeding, the milk supply in your breasts will decrease accordingly.

If weaning from the breast is postponed long enough, the baby may go directly to a cup, bypassing the bottles.

The baby might well be on three meals now with a fourth bottle at bedtime.

Fruit juices may be offered. The juice may be from a can of fruit that you eat if the fruit is canned in its natural juice and not in heavy syrup. The baby canned juices are too sweet and unnecessarily expensive. Juices can be diluted a bit with water, especially if baby refuses plain water. Such extra liquids should be given especially in hot weather and when baby is ill with a fever. So many babies get "rashy" from orange juice that it is advisable to start with some other kind. Orange juice should be avoided where there is a family history of allergy lest it sensitizes the baby.

SLEEPING

Babies begin to sleep through the night in different ways. One may drop the 2 A.M. feeding entirely by one month of age. Another may wake up for a feeding later and later each night. Some babies begin doing this with the 10 P.M. feeding, skipping it completely or waking up later and later. After three months of age, they may sleep through from 6 P.M. to 5 A.M.

Even after baby goes on four feedings a day, he may waken during the night occasionally and demand food. Feel free to give it to him without worrying that it will become a fixed habit.

As baby sleeps more at night, he is awake more during the day. His naps are reduced to four, then three and eventually two - the last usually when he is on three meals a day. Different babies will act differently.

SAFETY MEASURES

Now that baby is so much more active, you must be more careful than ever not to leave him anyplace from which he may fall. Don't turn your back for even an instant if you lay him on a sofa, bed, or any high place. Baby demands your full attention. You cannot do two things at once. Baby can wriggle out of an adult's arm if that person is trying to hold him with one arm and fix formula with the other. Put him down in the crib or playpen first.

Toys for baby should be too large to swallow and too tough to break. They should have no sharp points or edges. Select unbreakable plastic toys.

APPLIANCES TO SUIT BABY'S DEVELOPMENT

Now is a normal time to begin using a PLAYPEN. Since a baby of this age is awake much of the time, he should be taken from the confinement of his crib or bassinet into the relative freedom of the playpen. Here he can make his "swimming" motions on the firm pad and may also amuse himself by playing with a rattle or small stuffed toy.

Increasingly, child psychologists are taking a dim view of keeping a baby in a playpen for extended time periods, usually conceded to be an hour a day or more. Tactile and visual stimulation are far more important to baby's mental development at this age than previously thought. If you must put baby in a safe place for just a moment - enough time to answer the door, take a shower, or cook a quick meal - then using a playpen doesn't cut off his interactions enough to matter. But otherwise it is a good idea to allow baby the option of exploring a carefully baby-proofed house.

There are several styles of playpens from which to choose. Nearly all are folding types. Some are small enough for travel, such as the rather expensive net kind (this one, in particular, deprives him of much needed visual stimulation). As on a crib, the playpen bars should be no wider than two and three-eighths inches apart and, if wooden, without splinters. The sides should be 20 inches high and the floor capable of holding 80 pounds of static weights. There should be no sharp edges anywhere and the hinges should be non-folding.

Parents living in a small apartment may feel they don't have room for a playpen. In this situation, it is all the more important to set aside an area just for baby. Consider, too, that baby will be out of the playpen after he is walking well. So it is advisable to get a type that can be adapted later as a fence or gate at doorways and steps.

A SAFE FOLDING PLAY YARD

A baby of this age will not be able to sit up without some support for several months. It is difficult to prop him up for any length of time. A *stationary* JUMPER OR BOUNCE CHAIR may be used after the infant seat is outgrown. This is a canvas seat with two holes in front for baby's legs, built on a metal frame. It gives better support for the back and is far less dangerous than the hanging type of jumper with springs. babies get fatigued by the bouncing of the hanging type of chair and nearly always run the risk of tipping over in them or bouncing into the sharp corners of doorways. Babies who are ready to bear weight on their legs may enjoy some bouncing but they also need the type of leg exercises they get from attempts at crawling on the floor or playpen.

The baby is not yet ready for a HIGH CHAIR. As we shall discuss later, you may not even want a high chair but a safer, lower chair with table.

TOYS for handling and mouthing may be used even at this early age. Baby probably received many gift rattles and will now begin to enjoy them. Most are made of plastic and are well designed for these two purposes. You can also create some toys yourself, such as squeeze toys, made by sewing together toweling or oilcloth and stuffing with old cut-up nylon stockings. Stuffed toys do not have to be shaped like animals or dolls so you don't have to sew on buttons, either. A doughnut shape is more easily handled as well as mouthed by an infant of this age.

A CRADLE GYM is an attractive colored toy, usually made of plastic baubles. It can be tied to the side of the crib or hung on an elastic above it or attached to the playpen. You can make one yourself by fastening smooth objects to an elastic. Smooth plastic spoons, plastic bracelets, rattles, or any smooth surfaced toy too large to be swallowed may be used. Other material suitable for handling and chewing are plastic measuring spoons, a sponge and a floating bath toy. Your imagination will supply more ideas as you watch baby's development. Once baby starts pulling himself in the crib, remove any mobiles tied across or hanging above the crib.

Baby's other senses need stimulation, too, such as looking at bright colors and moving objects and listening to a variety of sounds. Baby may notice a brightly colored vase in a window with light coming through it. He may like TV too - in moderation - but remember that it is best not to have him face the brightness of the TV screen. Soft music from a radio, the rhythmic ticking of a clock, or a wind chime will all have their sound appeal. The sound baby likes best, however, is your voice as you talk, sing or hum to him.

CHECKUPS AND IMMUNIZATIONS

Baby will start getting his "shots" around two months of age and continue them at four and six months. The so-called basic series consists of three injections, two months apart, of a combination of diphtheria, pertussis (whopping cough) and tetanus (lockjaw). This combination is referred to as DPT. At two and four months, it is accompanied by polio vaccine by mouth. Measles vaccine is not given until 15 months of age.

You need not dread the "shots" for, although they hurt some, the baby at this age soon forgets them. Reactions to the present day vaccines are few and seldom severe. If the baby should be fussy after them, the doctor may allow you to give some acetaminophen. DO NOT give baby asprin.

Sometimes the immunization schedule is interrupted by little upsets or colds. But the interval between the administration of the basic series should not be overly long. The doctor will give you a record of what "shots" the baby had and what he needs next and when.

The importance of getting the full basic series is that the child should get a booster dose every few years. This "boosts" or increases his protection against these diseases much more than if he did not have the basic series. In the case of tetanus vaccine, for example, he can get a booster dose after a dirty wound, if he has had the basic series.

The American Academy of Pediatrics now recommends the newly licensed chicken pox (varicella) vaccine for universal use in early childhood, and for immunization in susceptible older children and adolescents.

A single dose should routinely be given between 12 and 18 months of age. This can be given at the same time as the child's first MMR (measles, mumps and rubella) immunization.

Once immunized, most individuals are protected from chicken pox. There has been no evidence of lost immunity after a six to ten year follow-up in healthy children. See page (86) for immunization chart.

THE DOCTOR'S EXAMINATION

HEIGHT AND WEIGHT. Your baby may have already grown three or four inches over his birth height and gained five or six pounds. His head may have grown as much as two inches in circumference. His brain is growing fast, too. The doctor will hesitate to compare your baby with any average height and weight chart because babies vary so much. It is better to compare your baby's height and weight with what it was the last time he was measured and weighed.

In contrast to the baby's appearance at birth, his whole body is now firm and well-rounded, assuming normal development, and the skin is clear. He may even smile up at the doctor. The doctor may hold a light or some other object above the baby and move it back and forth to see how well baby follows it with his eyes. At this age, the baby probably can follow the moving object clear over to the side, though he may prefer looking at the examiner's face. When some keys are shaken above the baby, he moves his arms and legs, too, as if he wishes he could hold them. When the keys are placed in his hand, he may grasp them briefly, then drop them.

HEAD. When the doctor pulls the three-month-old baby to a sitting position, the head may lag a little but is fairly steady. By four months, there will probably be no lag. The baby's head may be more shapely now and the front fontanelle a "finger breadth" smaller. The fontanelle may not close completely until from fifteen to eighteen months of age.

The eardrums are examined with an otoscope. They should be clear unless baby has a cold.

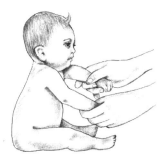

When you pull a three-month-old baby to a sitting position, the head should be steady

The throat is negative, little or no tonsils having appeared as yet. There may be some redness if baby has a cold.

CHEST. Rapid bone growth may show in small lumps along the baby's ribs. The doctor will examine these and also make sure you are giving enough vitamin D for growth and strength of all bones.

The doctor will listen with his stethoscope to baby's chest to check if the lungs are clear. The heart sounds and rhythm are checked, too. The heart rate is the usual rapid "tic-tac" rhythm of infancy. Incidentally, research suggests that a baby's chances of developing later respiratory or auditory problems are higher if one or both parents smoke. So if you or your partner are smokers who did not quit during pregnancy, now is a good time to thing seriously about it (see page 9).

ABDOMEN. This will feel soft to the doctor's examining hand. The navel is checked for any slight hernia. Some navels are so folded that they are not easy to cleanse. The doctor or the nurse may demonstrate the proper way of cleaning.

GENITALIA are checked for adhesions. If they and the rest of the diaper area show redness and irritation, the doctor will explain what to do.

FEET should be normal even though they look flat and have no arch.

As the climax to the examination, the first "shot" is given. Baby's surprised indignation should quickly pass.

CHAPTER 7

Your Baby Around Six Months of Age

THIS IS A PLEASANT time for you and the baby. He smiles a lot in response to your attentions. He even laughs out loud at antics. He can be content in the playpen for quite a while, playing with one toy. He is more sociable with you. But he may begin to be less so with outsiders. This is not fearfulness but discrimination on his part because he sees people better.

SIGNS OF DEVELOPMENT

The baby has been able to hold his head up well for a couple of months now. His vision has become keener. He can almost sit alone. He may sit with rounded back, leaning forward. He still needs support for his back. His hands and arms show the most remarkable development. He can reach and grasp with a "paw-like" grip. He can put something in his mouth and take it out again, look at it and pick it up again if he drops. At first, he reaches with both arms. In a short time, as he gains better control, he may use one hand

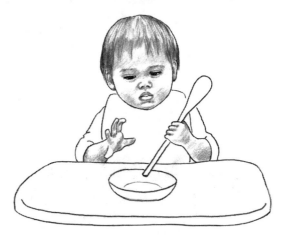

more than the other. Whether or not this indicates his future handedness remains to be seen. You can offer him a toy somewhat to the center and let baby decide which hand to use. He can get his foot to his mouth and frequently lies with feet in the air.

The age at which a baby will bear his weight standing when you hold him up varies a great deal. It is a matter of his ability to straighten his knees and then his hips. Be sure you are patient with him if he does not do it as soon as your neighbor's baby. Never accuse baby of "laziness" just because his legs seem "rubbery" for a longer time.

LANGUAGE

This, too, has its sequence of development in every child. In the beginning, baby's only language is crying, usually "Wa-a-a-a" and other vowels and a few consonant sounds, like k-, g-, and h- when he whimpers.

Around four months he might begin to babble, that is, repeat sounds. He also uses some of the lip-forming consonants, like m-, p-, and b-. He crows and squeals and babbles as if he were thoroughly enjoying the sounds he can make.

Language is very much a back and forth game. You learn quickly that different cries mean different things. Baby also learns to respond to your voice and the different tones you use, smiling at the pleasant tones and puckering at the "scolding" ones.

By six months he is making more non-crying sounds. He begins to use the tongue tip consonants, like d-, t-, and n-, thus adding more variety to his sounds. All this is important pre-language activity in which you can play a part.

FEEDING

Usually, by four to five months, the baby has developed the ability to swallow non-liquid foods. And by five to six months, he can show you if he wants or does not want food by leaning forward or leaning away.

Don't forget that all babies vary some, but most fall within this range. Most baby doctors recommend introducing solid foods at six months of age.

If so, do it gradually. One food type per week allows him to get used to the idea and build up good food habits. It also gives you a grace period in between to determine if baby has a negative reaction to something.

Infant cereals are a good place to start. They provide additional energy and iron and are easy to digest. Single grain cereals, especially rice, are the best. Three level tablespoons of electrolytic iron-fortified cereal diluted with breast milk or formula will do the trick. You may want to follow up with strained vegetables, fruits and meats (those prepared at home are just as nutritional as the commercial kinds and a lot cheaper). The order of introduction doesn't matter.

Be careful not to let the food stand for too long. Spinach, beets, turnips, or collard greens are bad choices because if they spoil, they can lead to some severe anemia problems.

Salt and sugar should not be added to commercial foods and you should not add them to anything you have prepared, either. Our over-dependence on such flavor enhancers is an acquired taste. If you can train baby early on not to use them beyond moderation, so much the better.

From now on, offer the baby more water. If possible, give it to him during feedings.

Although traditionalist have always counselled delaying the introduction of eggs, thinking nowadays has radically changed on the subject. By six months, a baby may be fed eggs if they seem to go down well.

If he has an allergic reaction to some foods, check with your doctor before eliminating them from his diet. Mistakes can be made, and the result is the elimination of valuable food.

Items with high allergy-related incidence, such as oranges, chocolate, and possibly fish, should not be given to the baby.

SLEEPING

The sleeping pattern shows progress, too. From six months on there are usually two naps a day, with the longer one in the afternoon, but this may vary. Since he is becoming more sociable, he may cry when you leave the room and also fuss at bedtime. You might find he will lie down more cooperatively if you rock him.

When is a baby tired? Many parents have observed about thumb-sucking, blanket-holding or hair-twisting that the baby only "does it when he is tired or going to sleep." Authorities assure us that these little traits are harmless. Yet they do worry mothers and fathers when they become fixed habits and persist into the pre-school years. Should they be nipped in the bud right now? The baby who seems to want extra sucking time can be allowed to have it whether on bottle, thumb, blanket or a pacifier. Try to develop this kind of philosophy about it. A baby may need these sources of rhythmic comfort from within himself. But as he develops and gets older, he should be able to derive more and more satisfaction from without, from people, toys and his surroundings. You can give him something else to hold in his hand, such as a toy, when he starts on his thumb.

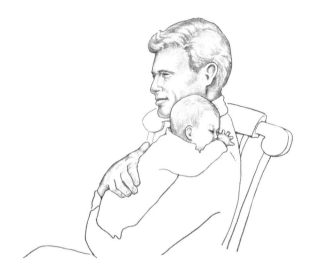

There are other more objectionable habits which some babies develop at bedtime which may begin soon after this age. These may be sitting and rocking or even head-banging. The significance of such behavior is not fully understood. If your baby starts either of these, you can try holding and rocking him yourself. Give him as much pleasant attention at bedtime as you possibly can.

APPLIANCES AND TOYS

For many parents, a PLAYPEN is almost a *must* now if you have not had it earlier. It is a well-protected place for baby to make all the motions he is practicing - the "swimming" that precedes crawling, the rolling over, or the lying with a toy rattle that is safe to handle and mouth. He should not be left in the playpen too long. He will be happier in it if you place it where he can see you at work.

If you are thinking in terms of a high chair, you might well consider one which can also be converted into a low chair. Or else get a low TABLE-SEAT combination. Accidents have happened with babies falling out of high chairs or sliding down and getting caught in the seat strap when left untended.

ROUNDED PLAYTHINGS of smooth wood or plastic make suitable and safe toys. They should be small enough to grasp but too large to swallow. Stuffed dolls or animals of cloth, plastic or rubber are also good, provided they have no removable parts, such as button eyes or squeaky whistles. Some things baby can have with your supervision are cloths and materials of interesting texture to feel and "scratch," as you will notice him doing. Paper which crumples with a satisfactory sound is fun, but must not be put in the mouth and swallowed. *Keep plastic bags away from baby*. Rounded rattles and rings are suitable for mouthing although the rattle should not have a long handle.

Baby might be intrigued by looking at himself in a MIRROR. One mother found she could keep her baby from squirming so much when she changed his diaper by propping a mirror alongside him on the bed.

The ability to reach and grasp is a great advancement in baby's development. He enjoys and learns so much from doing it that a mother or father should never slap a baby's hands in a mistaken attempt at early "discipline." The discipline needed now is on your part, mainly that you keep unsafe and fragile objects away from baby's reach.

> **Safety Measures**: Crib bumpers, stuffed animals and mobiles
> should be removed when baby starts pulling himself up with
> his hands. Put gates at top and bottom of every stairwell.

VISIT TO THE DOCTOR'S OFFICE

You will want to tell the doctor what the baby has been doing in the way of schedule and feeding and you may have a list of questions.

HEIGHT AND WEIGHT. By six months most babies have more than doubled their birth weight and lengthened out seven or eight inches. Since his three months checkup, your baby has probably averaged a gain in weight of two pounds per month and one half inch in height. The head and chest will have grown about one inch in circumference in the three to six months period.

GENERAL APPEARANCE. The doctor will feel the baby's arms and legs and look to see if the tissues are firm and the baby seems well-nourished. The fontanelle (soft spot) will have decreased in size.

Ears and throat are checked, particularly if there are signs of a cold or if there has been a recent respiratory infection.

Most exciting of all, a tooth or two - lower center - may be cutting through.

YOUR BABY AROUND THREE MONTHS OF AGE

Heart sounds are routinely checked. Breath sound are examined for possible harshness or wheezing. The abdomen is "palpated" when baby is not crying.

Diaper area rashes may show up now that baby is sleeping long hours at night without being changed.

The things baby is able to do will be a source of satisfaction to the examining doctor - head held up well, attempts at sitting briefly, and especially baby's use of arms and hands. Remember, progress is from the head downward, so don't expect much use of legs yet.

The third DPT concludes the basic series if baby has been able to have them all on time.

Baby may not need a routine checkup again until nine months. But, your doctor will tell you, call at any time, if necessary.

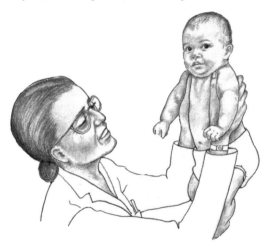

CHAPTER 8

Your Baby Around Nine Months of Age

THE EXCITEMENT OF WATCHING your baby grow never ceases. Each age brings forth its own special thrills. By nine months your baby has become a participating member of the family and may be included in many activities.

SIGNS OF DEVELOPMENT

The big achievement by this age is sitting up well, without any support. The baby probably enjoys sitting up and may object to lying down for a nap or even long enough to get his diapers changed.

Baby can do many more things with his hands now, such as holding his bottle, banging a toy, patting the table. He keeps reaching for objects. Try to surround him with safe things he can reach. And remove the others.

Not only can baby hold things well but he can release them and quickly make a game of dropping. Out of this comes his later ability to throw.

Finger development advances, too. He can pick up tiny things with thumb

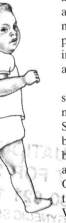

and forefinger. He may try to pick the flowers off a patterned cloth. This shows that his vision does not yet include a third dimension. When he can pull a toy towards himself by a string, he is observing the relationship of connected objects. He has accomplished a real engineering feat.

Use of the legs also progresses. After he sits, baby may get down on all fours and crawl or move around with some sort of hitching crawl. Some babies do not go through a crawling stage but go directly to standing and walking. Once baby starts to pull himself up in the crib, remove any mobiles tied across or hanging above the crib. Cover unused electrical outlets with safety caps or tape once baby starts walking or crawling. Walking however may not come about for several months yet.

54

The baby may do a nursery trick or two if taught, such as pat-a-cake or wave bye-bye. He responds more to people around him although he may show fear of strangers. This is part of his normal development because he can see farther and thus notices the difference in people. If the "stranger" will keep her distance for a while, he will soon be willing to make up to her.

LANGUAGE

Between four and nine months the baby's language is mostly babbling. Then he begins to combine sounds into syllables which he repeats. Out of this come the sounds Ma-Ma and Da-Da, which delight you both. It is your obvious pleasure and the fact that you repeat it back to baby that eventually make him associate these sounds with you. In this way language grows.

When he can make many sounds and also imitate conversational tones of voice, it is called "jargon." Very little, if any, is understandable. Jargon is important practice for baby and a fundamental part of pre-language development. Actual words come later and much more gradually.

FEEDING

Sometime after six months, most babies begin to take more interest in feeding and may want to do it themselves. Foods also require less straining. Simple mashing in some cases may be enough.

This is the period to begin with finger foods. These are foods which baby can safely hold by himself, perhaps put in his mouth, and gum down. Always keep an eye on him when he is eating finger foods and always peel fruits first. Never give him small, hard foods like raisins or nuts which could easily be aspirated on the way down. Teething biscuits and zwieback, however, are fine.

You may want to start the baby out on a training cup now, but don't expect instant success. Later on try a regular small cup, but don't put to much in it, "just fill cup half full." He may still want most of his liquids from the bottle. Don't be alarmed, he's not being babyish!

The spoon is a difficult implement to handle although baby may try. The active reaching and grabbing done at this age make it somewhat difficult to feed him. You can let him eat with a spoon until he gets tired or frustrated. Then take over. Or you might place a small shallow spoon in his hand. If his other hand interferes, give him another spoon or a toy to hold in it. Never tie the baby's hands down because they get in the way of feeding. Such things stifle development.

Baby will need his molar or grinding teeth before he can safely manage raw vegetables or some raw fruits. He will not be ready for these for a long time.

The baby's eating habits for the next few months are just plain "messy." He is constantly learning to be more expert. But this takes time, he is having fun even if you are not. As much as you may be looking forward to it, it may be better to postpone bringing baby to the family table for some "togetherness" at meal times. You could feed baby his supper first and let him have a crust of bread to mouth at the table and an empty cup to play with. Everyone may enjoy the meal more if you don't feed baby at the table just yet.

SLEEPING

Baby probably sleeps an average of fifteen hours a day, including his two naps. If he sleeps well through the night, be glad and get your own sleep for when he becomes a "ten-monther," he may not do so well.

ELIMINATION

This is not the time to start toilet training. If the baby has his bowel movements at a regular and hence predictable time, the mother might possibly catch the stool in a potty by holding the baby over it. This is not true "training," however. Most babies this age are not yet ready for training.

APPLIANCES

The playpen comes into its own now if baby is used to it. If you have not used a playpen previously, it is almost too late to start and expect baby to be happy in it. Baby can creep about safely in it and begin to pull himself up on its sides. Once up, he may feel stranded and not be able to let himself down. You can help him overcome this little fear by taking both hands and lowering him onto his seat with a gentle plop until he is willing to let go and do it himself.

A folding playpen is good for taking baby visiting. It will keep him away from the hostess's knickknacks. He can still be in the room and the center of admiring attention. He may prefer to take his nap in the pen instead of a strange bed.

SHOULD YOU BUY A WALKER?   According th the American Academy of Pediatrics, baby walkers should be banned and existing walkers destroyed to reduce infant injuries. The Academy says there is no scientific data to support claims that these walkers provide exercise, promote walking and keep babies quiet and happy. In 1993, there was a reported 24,000 walker-related injuries in children between the ages of 5 to 15 months.

Parents are sometimes "talked into" buying nursery equipment that is unnecessary and even dangerous. This is true of the walker. It does nothing for baby's development. It will not make him walk any sooner and may even delay his own efforts by hampering him from trying. Walking, as with other phases of his growth, is something the baby will do in his own good time. When his development is ready, nothing will stop a baby from walking. Until he is ready, nothing will speed it up either. He should not be accused of being "lazy" or not trying.

THE HIGH CHAIR VERSUS THE LOW CHAIR-TABLE. You are probably considering getting some kind of feeding chair for baby now. While the height of the standard high chair is convenient for you to feed the baby, it can be a hazard if baby falls or slides out of it. It does bring baby to the dining table as part of the family group but this might not be the ideal age for that.

Better than a high chair and usable for a longer period is a low chair-table combination. The table is like a small card table with a seat suspended in the middle of it. The seat can be folded in, making a complete table surface on which the child can play at a later age. At the present time, it offers baby a good chair with a back and a big tray surface around him. It will not be convenient for you to sit at and feed him, but it is a glorious place for him to feed himself and be messy.

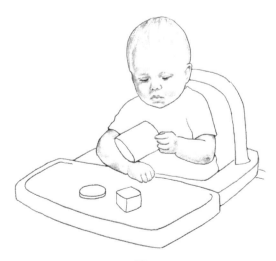

TOYS AND PLAY

All during childhood the stage of your child's development and his safety will determine what types of toys are best for him. There is too much tendency to buy something that appeals to an adult, such as an enormous stuffed animal so much bigger than the baby that he is afraid of it.

A baby at this age likes to handle blocks and bang them together. He also likes to put them into a big cup. Two-inch sized blocks are good and are suitable toys for a long time. He likes to put things into a basket and dump them out again. He loves to turn over wastebaskets. Why not see to it that there is nothing harmful in the wastebasket and then let him play with it? Nesting toys can also be used. All these activities will help baby get a concept of space. Pans, lids, plastic spoons and dishes found in every kitchen are other things that make adaptable toys. It is a good idea, however, to take these utensils out of the kitchen and bring them to baby rather than to allow him to be in the kitchen. He can be in his playpen watching you through the kitchen. From time to time you can offer the "treasures" to him.

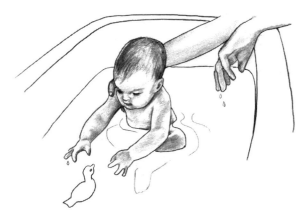

He will like a floating toy in his bath. He will enjoy playing in the water with a washcloth or sponge. Of course, you will never leave him unattended in the tub, even for an instant.

Some of the baby's triumphs are going to be a nuisance. For example, about this time baby will probably develop the ability to let go of an object and drop it. At first, it will most likely be his bottle. If his bottles are not already

58

of the plastic variety, you had better buy some to save breakage. A practical idea is to tie the bottle or a toy on to the edge of his tray or playpen with an elastic so that, instead of keeping you busy retrieving the object, he will learn to do it himself.

Talking and singing to baby, going to him frequently with a pat or hug, calling back to him when you go to another room are all good "games." They will help keep baby happy in his playpen as well as out. He will enjoy gentle roughhousing, such as bouncing and swinging.

There is still a strong tendency for baby to put things in his mouth. This must be taken into account when choosing his toys. No toy should have parts that are detachable or likely to be broken off.

Few toys need to be store-bought. Different sized cans may be used for a nesting set if the edges are smooth enough. You will find that baby loves to bite on his shoe. If you have an outgrown one, take the laces out of it, wash it and lo! - the baby has an improved teething ring.

VISIT TO THE DOCTOR'S OFFICE AT NINE MONTHS

At this checkup baby has probably gained three to four pounds over his weight at six months of age and may have grown one-and-a-half to two inches. The doctor may point out that growth is slowing down a bit, but is still fairly rapid, compared with what it will be in the next few years. You may be reminded that it is the rapid rate of growth that makes a baby have such a big appetite, and that as growth slows so will the food intake of the child. It's best to be warned in advance so you won't worry and think something is wrong if and when baby's appetite decreases.

If baby is standing or even walking while holding on to the crib rail or playpen rail or furniture, you might wonder whether or not it will injure baby's legs for him to stand on them so soon. The doctor will tell you that the baby may safely do anything he shows he is ready to do developmentally, providing adequate nutritional and vitamin requirements are met. In the days before vitamin D was given, babies did get bowed legs and other misshapen bones, not from walking too soon but from rickets caused by lack of vitamin D. It occurs much less often now because milks are enriched with vitamins A and D and because supplementary vitamins are also given.

Baby's feet and the way he stands and walks may look peculiar to you. A baby's foot looks flat because it is fat in the arch. The early walking is often imperfect, with a wide base and feet turned out for better balance. Minor difficulties may show up, such as feet or legs turning in or out. Ankles often appear weak and pronate, that is, bend inward. While the great majority of these things correct themselves after baby has become more expert at walking, they are certainly among the questions you will want to discuss with your doctor in the first months of walking.

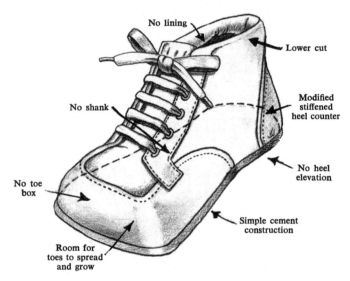

WHAT KIND OF SHOES TO BUY? Most doctors agree that baby doesn't need shoes before standing but that firm or moderately firm shoes may be purchased after baby begins to stand. They do not need to be high shoes. Indeed lower shoes may fit better in the heel, which is where the support is important.

About the only way to judge the fit of shoes is to measure the sole of one shoe on the sole of the opposite foot. Width should look adequate. Length should be not more than one-half inch beyond baby's toes. There is a tendency at some shoe stores to allow too much room for growth of a baby's foot so that the shoes are much too long at first. You can avoid this by doing the measuring yourself as described. Sometimes the shoes are so very stiff that you have to break them in by frequent bending of the sole.

The doctor may find things going so smoothly that baby will not need checkups so frequently. It cannot be emphasized too strongly, however, that you should keep in touch with the doctor if the situation calls for it.

CHAPTER 9

Baby is One Year Old!

BABY'S FIRST BIRTHDAY is a milestone. He himself will not be much different from what he was a month or so ago unless he has just started to walk. The big achievement of this age period is getting about, whether by walking or creeping. It opens a whole field of new experiences for the baby (not to mention mother and father).

Chances are baby has learned to pull himself to a standing position on the rungs of his playpen or some other furniture. He is likely to go through a stage of getting stranded up there and unable to let himself down until helped. Next he will walk holding on the furniture until brave enough to take off on his own.

He may become a creeper first, though not all babies do. He does this by going from a sitting position down on all fours or maybe "hitching" with one leg and arm in a sitting position. Even after he learns to walk, baby may get down and creep if he wants to go faster.

At first, baby's steps are wobbly. Falls are so frequent that he may have a constant bruise in the middle of his forehead. It's necessary to keep thing off the floor, for baby does not look where he is going and may stumble.

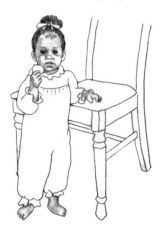

YOUR BABY IS ONE YEAR OLD!

Getting about is a great thrill. He is much less willing to stay in his playpen. It will be your job to make a larger "playpen" for him out of the whole room, removing fragile and forbidden objects and fencing off the rest.

Potential hazards are many. You have to become a safety "engineer," looking over the rooms several times a day, picking up and putting things away. It is important to learn what difficulties babies are likely to get into by reading reports and listening to experiences of others rather than by having bitter experiences of your own. Babies and pre-school children are inexperienced, heedless and rush headlong into anything. They are still incapable of being taught to mind much or to differentiate between forbidden objects and others. You must protect your little one until you can teach him. Concentrate on a safe house rather than on a pretty one.

SAFETY MEASURES

These are some of the things you *must* do and do *now*. Cover or fence off hot registers or stoves. Keep electric cords and appliances and all hot things out of reach. Get in the habit of turning pot handles inward on the stove. Use table mats instead of tablecloths. Baby may think he can pull himself up on a tablecloth and instead brings things crashing down on himself. Tie up any loose, dangling telephone cords.

The cupboard under the kitchen sink (a most attractive place for a baby of this age) should have a lock on it if cleansers, detergents, bleaches or furniture polish are kept there. It is better to keep baby out of the kitchen. Always keep him away from any area in basement or garage where paint, kerosene products, or pesticides are stored.

As soon as you use medicine of *any kind*, replace the cap and put the bottle out of reach, preferably locked up. You can't depend on the so-called "safety" cap now used on some baby medicines. Toddlers are smart enough to open them. And if the cap hasn't been put back, he doesn't even have to try.

Safety covers can be bought to cover up electric sockets when not in use and thus keep prying little fingers out.

These precautions are listed again in the chapter on "Poisoning and Accidents" but they need to be stressed, particularly when the child is beginning to get about and into things. Since the baby is incapable of taking much discipline at this age, the discipline must be yours. You have to train yourself to go over the house each day or more often until it becomes second nature. When you take baby visiting to Grandma's and Grandpa's, you will have to ask her to do the same. If she says, "But this child must learn to mind!", your

YOUR BABY IS ONE YEAR OLD!

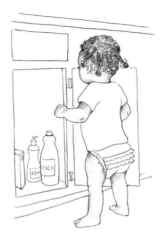

KEEP IT LOCKED!

answer can well be "Since he is so little and inexperienced, I want to start out by making it easier for him to obey."

It is said that baby learns more in his first year than in the rest of his life. While "learning to mind" is important, it need not be the only important thing. Baby must also learn much about the nature of the world around him. If you are constantly saying "No-No" or slapping his hands, you will stifle this great creative urge to learn. It's true he understands what "No-No" means. Before long he will be using it himself to your dismay. If it is applied to too many of his activities, he will get the idea that they are all bad. A more positive approach, and one which is much more challenging to you, will be to use "No-No" only for important things, such as possible hazards. Then it means much more to him. Whenever you forbid baby from doing something, give him something else to do instead. This requires ingenuity. What you have him to do may be very simple. When you go visiting, for example, you may take his favorite toy and bring out one every time he heads for the host's possessions. Gently but firmly taking away a forbidden object, saying "That's the lady's," is better than shouting "No-No." Baby himself should be removed from a scene of too many temptations and settled in a better spot.

YOUR BABY IS ONE YEAR OLD!

FEEDING

By one year of age the baby is on coarser foods. He can take many foods from the family table if they re not in large pieces. He cannot really chew until he gets his molar (double) teeth. He will be more choosy about his foods and should be allowed some freedom of choice. Tasty preparation will help his appetite just as it does the rest of the family. Baby canned food is pretty flat-tasting. It can be made more palatable by using it in recipes, as vegetables in soups and fruits in puddings. Very mild custard-type puddings are the best forms in which to feed egg. Cooking renders eggs more digestible and less allergenic. Do not offer nuts, popcorn or raw vegetables.

The baby will not be able to manage a spoon well by turning it over at the proper time for about six months yet. He may let you help him guide it to his mouth or even take over the spoon feeding at the end of the meal when he is tired.

SLEEPING AND DRESSING

If he resists going to sleep, it is because he does not want to be separated from people and his new activities. Bouncing play is fine, but better not just before bedtime lest baby becomes over-stimulated and more reluctant to sleep. Two naps are still usual.

He may cooperate a little in getting dressed by holding still. Up till now, it probably has been a struggle to dress that "wiggler."

TOYS

Push and pull toys are suitable for this age. These add zest to walking, especially if they make noise. Blocks of two-inch square size are easy to handle. The things the baby progressively does with them show the development of his mind and muscle coordination. At one year he tries to combine two blocks and likes to put them in a cup and dump them out again.

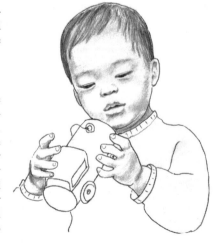

He likes to empty wastebaskets and pull books out of shelves. His own books can be put on a low shelf which is easy for him to reach. Other books should be put out of reach. Baby will look at pictures in a book if you name them, but he will prefer to take the book apart. Don't be cross. He is simply learning the nature of paper and books, not just being destructive.

Windup and complicated toys have no place yet. A windup toy is soon broken. Baby will get more pleasure out of a toy he can push or pull himself. A very simple block train with notches to put the cars together is far better at this age than metal or plastic cars with wheels. The latter may not be safe if baby falls on sharp or broken edges. Train tacks are not advisable for years yet. Things to feel, mouth, suck, bite, pat, put in, take out, drop, roll - all are acceptable. Every toy given to baby should be smooth and unbreakable, chewable but too large to be swallowed or choked on and should not have any small removable or breakable parts.

SPEECH

First words are uttered at about one year of age. But many of his sounds will still be unintelligible jargon. You can use many words to him which he will come to understand before he utters them himself. Use *names* of things frequently. Sentences and explanations will only confuse him. For the next six months he will be more interested in getting around than in learning to talk.

HABITS AND EMOTIONS

Thumb-sucking frequently drops out by the first birthday except when baby is tired or cross. If it lasts much longer, it is often accompanied by some activity of the other hand, such as fondling or picking at a favorite blanket or stuffed animal or twiddling his hair. We do not know the significance of this common phenomenon but it does seem to give great comfort to some children. It may continue considerably longer than the first birthday. Forcible removal of such a blanket or interruption of such a habit may distress the child greatly. When these habits persist into the preschool years, they may be an indication that the child needs more comfort and affection from those around him.

Emotions develop, too. such as anger, fear, jealousy, anxiety and frustrations. This is "progress?" "He never did *that* before!" you will exclaim. Yes, they are as much a part of normal development as are affection and some of the more pleasant emotions.

Temper tantrums appear, too. Even these are part of normal development. The first temper tantrum will most likely take you by surprise. It also takes baby unawares. He may be as amazed as you at his own sudden surge of anger, a new feeling. How will you handle this situation? Assuredly not by punishment, for in a sense he cannot help it. Punishment would only add to his anger.

If the tantrum is very severe (sometimes they may lead to breath-holding and even turning blue), you may have to hold baby until it passes. Then try by any means except punishment to show the child that there are better ways of getting what he wants. some tantrums may be headed off by a more gradual approach when taking away something from the child or by giving a little warning time before taking him off to bed. Don't let baby get over-tired before you take him to bed or his fatigue will make him extra irritable. Like other phases of development, tantrums too will pass if handled wisely.

TOILET TRAINING

To many persons, one year of age seems like such a milestone that they think they must immediately get busy with toilet training. Most babies, however, are not yet ready for it. Remember that development always comes about in a certain order. First the child holds his head up before he can sit; then he sits before he can stand, and so on. These things are well-known. But is is not generally recognized that a child's capacity for toilet control does not come until after he starts to walk. Since the age of walking is so variable, it is reasonable that the age for accepting toilet training will also vary. There have been instances of babies, usually girls, being trained early. Some children, usually boys, may be two years old or more before being completely trained. In some cases, it seems to come about easily and without effort on your part. In many instances it is more gradual and goes through stages as described in the next chapter.

You will need some special seat for the child. It is not too early to get that, showing the child that it is to be his own. Since it is difficult to know whether a potty chair or a seat on the toilet will work best for your child until you try, there is something to be said for a borrowing system. It seems to delay training efforts to expect a child to use the big toilet without any modifying seat.

The next two chapters will give suggestions and recommendations for toilet training.

SHOULD BABY HAVE A BIRTHDAY PARTY?

You will notice in the pictures that appear in the newspapers of one-year-old parties that some children are usually crying. There is too much noise and confusion and their usual routines are upset. Babies of this age like attention from adults but do not appreciate each other. They are likely to push and pull and poke each other like inanimate objects. Have your party but make it brief and not at nap time. Keep these limitations in mind in planning any social affairs.

BODY GROWTH DURING THE FIRST YEAR

By his first birthday, the baby has probably tripled his birth weight, grown one third again of his birth length and his head and chest have increased about one third of their birth circumference. He is likely to have six or eight teeth, all front incisors, although teething is quite variable.

Between nine and twelve months, baby should be tested for tuberculosis.

CHAPTER 10

Your Baby Around Fifteen Months

BY THIS AGE YOUR baby will probably be walking. Remember that some are normally slower in doing so. This new ability brings baby a sense of power that he thinks he can do anything. He tries to do too much too vigorously. He enjoys his own actions and changes of positions so much that he wears himself out. He gets frustrated not only by your "No-No's" but also at his own inability to do things. He may frequently cry and even have temper tantrums. At such times he needs to be picked up or provided with quieter activity.

Crawling gets a baby around pretty fast, too. Whatever the means of locomotion, the baby becomes an explorer of everything. Drawers, cupboards and doors are opened and shut. Wastebaskets are used to put in and take out of, or put in and dump. Handles and knobs are turned, twisted and broken off. If baby comes across a fragile, breakable or tearable object, he will pull it apart.

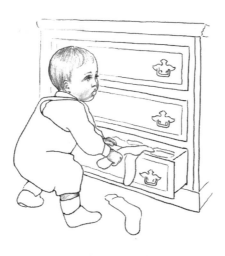

YOUR BABY IS ONE YEAR OLD!

Baby is a bundle of energy. Push, pull, bang and pat. Pick up and drop. Look at his smile of satisfaction as he lets something drop from a height. Touch and feel, not only with his hands and fingers but with mouth and lips. The lips are even more sensitive to touch than the fingers. Then there is that extra sensation of taste.

EATING

At this age baby may eat almost everything except raw vegetable, nuts and popcorn, berries with large seeds, candy because it is too sweet, and coarse foods like bran cereals because they irritate the intestinal tract. Avoid much spiciness in foods and strongly flavored vegetables, such as brussel sprouts or onions.

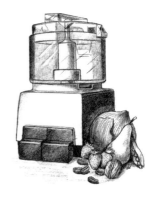

Meat is important as a source of protein ("growing food") and iron. Even with few teeth baby can manage meat, put through a food processor, or well-stewed meat if meat has been trimmed and finely chopped. There are canned baby "sausages" which he may like. Junior food meats are good, too.

The spoon is still a complicated tool for him. He has to fill it, get the food to his mouth and then turn over the spoon in his mouth. This last ability may be perfected about now but he needs practice to learn the technique. Give him finger foods like a piece of cooked carrot, chunks of hamburger, even French fried potatoes cut in half. Then let him try the spoon foods. After he gets tired or frustrated with the spoon, baby might let you give him a few spoonfuls with another spoon while he holds on to his own. When he is tired or ill, he may like to be fed "like a baby" again.

Fruits are generally liked, vegetables often disliked. To a certain extent, you can substitute one for the other. There is still nutritional merit in giving green and yellow vegetables, but both need not be given every day. Usually you can find one vegetable or method of preparation he likes. Depend on this until he takes more variety.

A BALANCED DIET FOR BABY

A balanced diet, as you learned during pregnancy if not before, consists of the following classes of food:

PROTEINS, OR "BODY-BUILDING FOODS." These are mainly meat, fish, cheese, eggs. Milk has been baby's main source of protein. He does not need so much now that he is on more solid foods. It may be given as ice cream and used in cooking. Cheese can be used in cooked dishes that the family eats or as chunks of finger food. Eggs should always be cooked, never given raw. If boiled eggs are disliked, they may be more acceptable scrambled with a little milk or used in the custard type desserts which are not too sweet.

CARBOHYDRATES, OR "ENERGY FOODS." Baby can have bread in the form of toast, zwieback, bread sticks, teething biscuits and simple non-crumbly cookies like the arrowroot which are not very sweet. Candy is too concentrated a form of sugar for his teeth. It is better for him to get accustomed to less sweet foods. Some of the new sugared dry cereals are not too sweet and may please him as finger food that will keep a baby busy for hours.

FRUITS AND VEGETABLES supply minerals, vitamins and bulk to the diet although there is some calorie value, too.

FATS are obtained from whole (homogenized) milk and a little margarine or butter. Nutritionally, the latter are equal.

VITAMINS. Many foods are enriched with vitamins and iron. Real vitamin deficiencies are seldom seen these days. It is customary to supplement a baby's diet with vitamins ABC and D or AD and C for the first two years because rapid growth increases the requirements. This is especially so if the mother is breastfeeding and if the baby lacks sunlight because of the winter weather. There is no advantage in the so called "natural" vitamins though food faddist may try to tell you so. It is never necessary to supplement with minerals if the diet is adequate.

FLUORIDE has a definite protective effect on forming teeth. It should be given from an early age, if it is not in the public water supply. It is perfectly safe.

Mothers were probably instructed to eat some of these food substances from each group every day for a balanced diet during their prenatal period. But will baby "balance?" A 15-monther is seldom in this kind of balance. He may relish fruit one day and will have nothing to do with it the next. He refuses his milk for a week, his solids the next. At dinner he might eat one thing as if he could never get enough and refuse everything else. Instead of trying a new food, he clamps his mouth shut and pushes it away. The only kind of balance he shows is an up and down see-saw of likes and dislikes. In your panic and bafflement, you may try to force him to eat the things you know he must have, which only makes matters much worse.

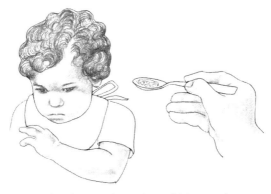

There are a couple of reassuring points which your doctor can give you at this stage for you will surely ask for advice. No doubt, you will be told that as baby's growth slows down so does baby's intake of food. He does not need so much food as he did several months age. The other point is that while he will not get a balanced diet every day, he is likely to achieve a balance over a longer period of days and weeks, even with this hit-and-miss type of eating. No baby has ever been known to starve under these conditions although is is hard to convince parents of that.

Then, too, there are so many other things that baby would sooner do than eat. He never sits still. On occasion you may even have to feed him standing up! Well, why not?

Real appetite problems of the pre-school period may result from poor handling of this period. There is nothing more destructive to a child's appetite than to have adults watch every bite he does or does not put into his mouth and try to force more food on him than he wants or needs.

In a relaxed family atmosphere it is nice to have the baby at the table. He may even eat better in imitation of others. If the excitement distracts him from eating and especially if people pay too much attention to his eating or criticize his imperfect manners, then it is better for him to eat by himself, at least for part of the meal. At some ages a young child definitely eats some of his meals better by himself. Parents are the best judges of this or may find out by trying it both ways.

71

YOUR BABY IS ONE YEAR OLD!

After warning you and possibly making you dread a feeding problem, you may not have it at all. If you are among those wise parents who manage a baby with an air of calm expectancy that he will eat well and go to sleep at regular times, you will have far fewer problems. You may also be more observant of developmental changes in your child and consequently go along with them better. These are some of the "secrets" of parents of well-behave children.

SLEEPING

Baby gets tired after his hectic activity. But he does not realize that sleep is what he needs. It will be a long, long time before he will admit "I am tired." His behavior will signal this to you at least several times a day. Parents and grandparents, too, may regard a cranky, disobedient child as "bad" when he is merely tired. Even when worn out, baby does not want to leave all his fascinating new activities and go to bed. He will eat when hungry, drink when thirsty, but not go to bed very willingly even when tired. At this age a little warning before he has to go to bed is helpful. It may prevent his objections or even a tantrum. You can lead up to bedtime gradually by getting baby into his pajamas and telling a story before the inevitable. Some clever parents can manage this simply by assuming a confident air that baby will go to bed.

Night sleep averages twelve to thirteen hours once baby is in bed. The sleep may be disturbed, however, especially if the last part of his day had been hectic. Comfort baby if he wakens, but do *not* take him into your bed or then he will never want to stay in his own.

TOYS AND PLAY

Baby won't stay in his playpen now, at least not much. You should have made the whole room into a larger, safe play area. The best of rooms prepared in this way is still likely to have some unremovable or forbidden objects in it which will give baby plenty of opportunity to find out what things are. And don't deliberately tempt him with things just to teach him discipline. TV knobs are too tempting to resist and often get broken. Such temptations are better fenced off, making it easier for the baby to mind, as well as saving the TV.

Fortunately, a child of this age is easily distracted by something else. You should find substitute things he can do. One father, for instance, noticing that his child liked to fiddle with a lock, went to a hardware store and got one which he mounted on a light board for the child to play with. Indeed toys like this can be bought. You can also make your own "Busy Boxes." Although a home-made toy is cruder in form, it would be much mor meaningful both to you and your baby because you have observed what your baby can do and likes to do. A mother whose child was fascinated by buttons and buttonholes gave the child an old coat with big buttons and buttonholes to play with.

Other home-made toys may be constructed from different sized milk cartons. A shoe box with a slot in the cover makes a fine 'mailbox." since picture books are likely to be expendable, you can make pictures for baby by patting bright cutouts on a cardboard. As he begins to talk, he will point to the pictures and name the objects. He will like the bright, even garish, colors better than subdued pastels. He may already have push or pull toys to help has balance in walking.

SOCIAL ACTIONS

With his mother and father the baby alternates between dependence and independence. He cannot wait to get down from her lap and get going, though not too far. He soon comes back to check on her whereabouts.

Baby may still be wary of strangers. If the visitor who rushes over and hugs him on arrival would only stay across the room for awhile and be looked over, she would be much better liked. Hide-and-seek and closing his eyes at strangers are baby's sort of "power" plays. Do they not make people disappear? Once acquainted, baby is quite willing to "show off" and be an entertainer.

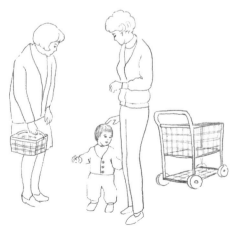

YOUR BABY IS ONE YEAR OLD!

SPEECH

If there are people around, especially children whose chief joy it is to bring him things, baby may not need to bother with words. He will point or use one word or sound for many things. Tell older children to use a name every time they bring baby anything. Do the same yourself. Never offer him anything silently.

From now until the end of the second year, baby will be much more interested in walking than in talking. He adds only a few words to his vocabulary. Jargon makes up most utterances. It is a "rehearsal" for later clear speech.

Keep in mind that, even if baby does not talk much or clearly, he is continually listening. His speech is more likely to be clear later on if you enunciate clearly now.

TOILET DEVELOPMENT AND PARENT TRAINING

No, we did not get our signals mixed in this heading. We do not like the term "training" in connection with toilet control. It implies that it is a matter of discipline *which it is not*. It is rather a matter of development, development of the child's ability to control his urinating and bowel movements and a complex balance of holding and releasing. The age at which the child achieves such control is extremely variable. As a rule girls are earlier than boys.

Control comes in stages. The child who points to a puddle he has made has taken the first step by being aware that he has wet. It may be quite a time before he is aware ahead of time that he needs to go. But he may give signals to that effect so that his mother or father can put him on the toilet. Such signals can be pulling at pants, grunting or even squatting. If the parent is keen enough to catch these signs, the child can be put on the toilet or potty chair and the urine or bowel movement "caught." This is parent training, not yet child control.

The next step in developing control may be very disturbing and even bewildering to the parent. This is when the child is placed on the potty, possibly has even signalled, but does nothing until right after getting off! This happens to so many children that it must almost be regarded as a normal stage of development. Do you remember how hard it was for you to use the bedpan the first few times in the hospital? You just couldn't seem to void until you got into an accustomed position on a toilet. So it can be with the child. He is accustomed to going in his diapers in a standing or even squatting position or maybe just sitting on the floor. His first times over an unaccustomed opening are like your first time with a bedpan.

74

Continue to encourage the baby to be comfortable having the potty chair around. You may even want to put it into his room, in a corner somewhere. Tell him what it is meant for and maybe sit him on it (possibly with his diaper still on). But, above all, don't rush or pressure him into anything.

A TYPICAL CHECKUP AT FIFTEEN MONTHS

Here is an example of what occurred when one baby girl, Angie, went in for her fifteen month examination.

Angie's mother was glad to have the baby get a checkup at this time for she was running into a feeding problem. Angie refused to drink her milk or touch any vegetables. She was on a hamburger jag, refusing most other foods. When her mother found that Angie had gained only one pound in three months, she became very worried.

The doctor assured the mother that this kind of "trouble" was normal for this age. He said Angie was in the middle of her normal growth (she had grown an inch in the three months) and weight curve. He advised that she offer the baby some choices at every meal even if it did seem wasteful when she did not "clean up her plate." He warned the mother against falling into the "trap" of trying to force food or nagging at Angie for not eating. He didn't even like discussing the problem in front of the child. He was sure she was taking it all in. Young children, he said, often find they get more attention by not eating and exploit it for all it is worth since they like attention better than food.

On his examination, he found Angie to be progressing well. She was adequately nourished, had no signs of illness and was walking fine.

You might be interested in using Angie's case history as a basis of comparison with your own child's development. But always bear in mind that each child is different.

CHAPTER 11

Your Baby Around Eighteen Months

THE BABY LOOKS MORE grown up now, even though he has probably not grown very much in height since one year of age; maybe about three inches. His weight may also be fairly stable. He may not have added much more than a few pounds.

PHYSICAL DEVELOPMENT

Motion-wise, he walks rather stiffly. He can run, though awkwardly. He can't run around corners yet. He might be able to walk upstairs with help. Walking down is more complicated. There is one big advance. He not only can climb into a chair, he can push the chair and then climb into it, thereby opening up a number of dangerous fields of exploration. (At the Poison Control Center, parents have frequently been heard to say, "But I never knew he could climb so high!") One has to be mighty alert to keep one jump ahead of a baby's development.

Baby is getting pretty good at throwing, too. He may even be able to throw a ball overhand, though not aim it. Even before his aim develops, you can begin showing your little one that rocks should never go towards people and animals, but away from them. Then, contradictory as we are, we show the child how to aim a ball at a person! Well, there is a simple lesson in this. The child learns the difference in aiming balls and rocks. With enough time and repetition, the ideas get across. You are the one to find out at what age these lessons can be learned by your child.

EATING

The baby may be eating less because his growth is slowing down. It may take him several months to gain a pound. For awhile his weight almost seems stationary. Then he goes through a spurt of growing and gaining. But nothing like the rapid rate of the first year will ever be achieved again. Taking a cue from this, you could offer smaller servings so he can have the satisfaction of cleaning up his plate. Do not insist, however, that he finish everything. If he begins cutting down on milk too much (a pint or so is enough now), you can make it up with bits of mild cheese, cottage cheese, creamed dishes and creamed soups, milk on puddings and cereals, and ice cream.

Meat is important for body building and as the main source of iron. Enriched cereals and breads also contribute some iron. If the baby likes only only one kind of meat, let him have it every day. Some meat can be cut up into a sort of julienne strip and used as finger food, which he will enjoy. Fish can be given but you must be extremely careful to remove the bones. Eggs are much less important than meat.

The child is entitled to some likes and dislikes just as you are. He is also entitled to well-cooked food. You cannot pass off on baby some left-over meat or barely warmed baby food from a can without any seasoning. Admittedly, it is discouraging to cook a meal and have a fussy child refuse to eat it. But if it is tasty and you have an air of assurance that he will eat and if the atmosphere at the table is pleasant, appetite problems do not occur so often. Also, the good smell of cooking makes any appetite better.

The long aim of having your child form good eating habits, including a balanced diet, and liking his food is much more important than getting in a certain amount of foods or certain kinds of food every day.

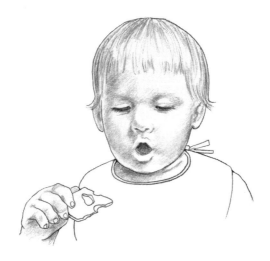

The right tools and dishes help, too. A baby can grasp a broad, short, straight handle on a spoon. The bowl of a spoon should be wide as well as long so he can get it into his mouth sideways. At this age he begins to get the idea of turning over the spoon in his mouth at the right time. His plate should be a shallow bowl so he can push against the sides with his spoon. One mother said her little girl managed a fork better and earlier than a spoon because she could spear with it. Such a baby fork should have blunt points and a short straight handle like the spoon.

A cup that has a handle big enough for the child to put his hand through is an aid when he begins to pick it up with one hand. A rather shallow (and less tippable) cup is good.

SLEEPING

Sleep averages thirteen hours, with one daytime nap. At night baby may awaken at times. He only needs a little comfort and reassurance, or changing, which should be done in his bed.

PLAY ABILITY

The child of this age can handle balls of different sizes. A medium sized, lightweight one for rolling, throwing or bouncing and possibly a big beach ball to roll around on for fun. These help to develop both small and large muscles.

A low-seat of nontippable, non-movable steps would be fine to have outdoors for the child to use in his constant climbing.

Does he like better to push or pull? One thing he will prefer is to push his carriage or go-cart instead of riding in it. He may have a wheeled toy that makes a noise when he pulls it. He will like a toy telephone and "use" it in a comically grown-up manner. Time for another simple lesson: the real telephone is not to be played with. Better get the telephone cord out of reach of grasping hands and stumbling feet, too.

Blocks are good playthings for many ages. Right now your child may be able to build up a small tower out of two-inch kindergarten blocks. Developmental tests show that to pile one on top of the other, the child has to be able to let go of a block with some accuracy. Blocks can be of different sizes, shapes and colors. Later he will learn his colors from them. Now he learns a lot by handling different sizes and shapes.

He needs to learn about textures, too. Give your child a chance to play with soft and hard things, fuzzy and cuddly toys, rough and smooth objects, firm and runny substances. Water, sand, mud are all things he wants to feel

DIET SUGGESTIONS

Food	How Often	Remarks
Meat	Once a day	
Chicken or Fish	Occasionally, in substitution	
Cooked vegetables	Once a day	May be green or yellow, mashed for practice with spoon, or in pieces for finger food. Yellow vegetables, such as carrots, given too often can cause yellow color in skin, called *carotenemia*.
Fruit	Once or twice a day	May be canned, pureed, mashed or finger food.
Egg (cooked)	Two or three times per week	Also in puddings.
Cereal (cooked or flakes)	Once a day	
Toast, non-crumbly crackers, zwieback		Margarine, peanut butter or jelly allowed, *in moderation*.
Milk	With all meals or between meals	A pint or more a day in any form.
Soups		If nourishing, such as vegetable, potato or creamed. Non-spicy canned soups acceptable.
Potatoes	Two or three times per week	Baked potato is best.
Gravy		Only if it helps with intake and is not greasy. Does not have nutritive value of meat.
Fruit juices	Between meals	As a snack. Need not be citrus. Canned juice acceptable.
Desserts		Simple puddings, plain cookies, ice cream. Avoid cake, pie, candy and especially nuts and popcorn.

and play with . . . sometimes even his own bowel movement. This may be a very upsetting experience to you. Keep in mind that to the child it is only another substance to explore. There is nothing in his past background to tell him that it is "nasty" or "bad."

Now he can help turn the pages of a book. He may even be able to point out some of the pictures. His memory is developing as shown by his knowing where things are, where they were and where they belong. Since he can also obey simple commands, these new abilities can be made use of to begin to teach him to put his toys away. A set of low shelves works better than a box. Or if you can give him a low cupboard of his own, he can have the fun of opening and closing the cupboard doors which he has been trying to do to your cupboards until you have had to lock them.

SPEECH ABILITIES

Jargon is at a peak. He may use about ten or twelve words but understands and responds to many more. For instance, he can point to his face and body features when you ask him. Next he will use some words that describe the world outside himself.

It cannot be stressed enough that the child will eventually speak more plainly if he hears clear, distinct speech. In one family where all the children seemed to have speech defects, the father did not realize how very blurred and hurried his own speech was. Each child in turn imitated the others.

While he can understand many words, he will not yet understand much in the way of explanations. Instead of telling the child why he cannot do certain things, it is more effective to pick him up and remove him from them, or distract him with something else. Whenever possible, try to make the transition to something else gradual. This will help to avoid some temper tantrums. To keep a child from touching a forbidden object, you can say "That's Mommy's," or "That's hot!" This would be the extent of his understanding of any explanations. You should put most forbidden things away.

SOCIABILITY

Baby is still completely self-centered. A child of a year-and-a-half is so absorbed in his own activities that he does not even mind the arrival of a new baby in the family as much as he would later, say at three years. But he would mind having to give up his bed to the newcomer. That would be too much.

The child of this age is only beginning to understand social relationships. He will still poke and push other babies. His sense of possession will be very strong for the next months. He cannot be expected to share for some time. If another child of the same age comes to visit, you had better put away prized toys that are likely to be fought over. Or else supply duplications.

TOILET CONTROL

Tommy's parents decided that Tommy was going to be toilet trained before the family went on vacation. Tommy was about one year old at this time. Vacation was two months off. Tommy was put on a potty chair every hour during the day and made to sit there until he "went". Tommy's parents were business executives who thought they could apply job training methods to their child. Yet they would never think of trying to make Tommy walk by putting him up on his feet every hour and saying "Go." They knew Tommy would walk when ready and could not be hurried into it. The doctor had to point out to these parents that the child also has to be ready for toilet training before much can be accomplished.

Tommy's parents were pretty sure that he knew what was wanted of him. He was a bright, alert child. When he wouldn't go, this was termed "stubbornness." Sometimes he would sit on the potty chair for awhile and then go right after he was allowed to get off. Then he was accused of being "spiteful". By this time relationships between child and parents had deteriorated badly, resulting in a visit to the doctor's office for advice.

Many adults make the same mistake. One has to wait on development of control over the sphincter muscles around the rectum and bladder outlets before beginning training. These do not mature until after the child begins to walk - which means an average range from eighteen to twenty four months. Remember, "average" means some will be younger and some as late as three years of age before they are able to accept training. The child may "know" well what is expected of him and still not be able to comply because of later development.

How can you tell when your child is ready? For one thing, he has made a giant sep toward control when he can stay dry for as long as two hours and wakes up dry from his nap. He surely cannot last much longer, so you put him on the potty when you think he can go. But not for more than a minute or so. And not more often than every two hours, or whatever you find his interval of staying dry to be. If he goes, fine. If not, take him off and allow him to play a while. Whenever he is on the potty, use some word or sound that he will be able to connect with going. "Potty" seems to come naturally to many parents. The same word covers both wetting and bowel movements. Later on, you can use different words or sound for each when he is able to tell which it is he has to do.

Bowel control tends to precede bladder control. If the bowel movements are at regular times, you may be able to "catch" them by putting him on at those times. You know yourself that you can move your bowels only when you have the urge. But we illogically expect a child to have his bowel movement at our convenience. Do not use suppositories or enemas to bring this about. It tampers with the natural urge which may be at irregular times and still be normal.

If you have become tense and anxious about toilet training, it will be more difficult to achieve. A child may need to go and still tighten up as soon as he is put on, just as we do occasionally. It is a new and unaccustomed position to him. The child may be more comfortable and relaxed on a potty chair with his feet on the floor. Or a seat on the big toilet may suit him better. This needs a footrest for it is hard to evacuate with legs dangling. Steps in front of the big toilet are necessary for the child to get up on the seat easily. He should also be able to take his pants off easily. This means using training pants rather than diapers. Some mothers find that letting the child run around without pants before the expected bowel movement makes him "go" more readily. The main point is that almost any method works if the child is ready. Nothing works if he is not ready.

A potty chair has the advantage of movability from room to room but has the disadvantage of being closer to the floor and, thus, uncomfortably cold. After all, nothing is sacred about the bathroom for such purposes. A potty chair can also be taken on trips for the baby so his "training" will not be interrupted. A boy's potty chair should have a urine deflector.

CHECKUPS AND BOOSTERS

Eighteen months is a good time for a checkup. The doctor may show more interest in your child's walking and general development than in a detailed physical checkup, if the child seems well.

Booster immunizations are due for DPT and polio, if the basic series was completed a year ago.

In observing your own child, try to differentiate developmental stages and characteristics from mere naughtiness. You will then find yourself able to give the child guidance rather than to administer punishment. You will be able to help him from one stage to the next by anticipating what is to come. This is why it is important to understand child development. The more you understand your own child, the better a parent you will be.

CHAPTER 12

The Importance of Immunization

SOME DISEASES HAVE BEEN preventable by vaccination programs for such a long time that the diseases have become rarities. These include smallpox, diphtheria and whooping cough. TETANUS VACCINE is customarily included with diphtheria and whooping cough as a three-in-one shot or DPT given in three doses in early infancy. "Booster" DPT is given at eighteen months and four years.

New recommendations made by the American Academy of Pediatrics (AAP) to all member pediatricians was reported in the December 1998 issue of the AAP's official news magazine. The AAP now recommends that most children in the USA receive the inactivated polio virus vaccine (IPV) which should be given by an injection, at 2 and 4 months of age for the first two doses. Either the IPV or the oral polio virus (OPV) is recommended for the third dose at 6 to 18 months and the fourth dose at 4 to 6 years.

The inactivated polio vaccine only is recommended for immunocompromised (persons with a weakened immune system) and their household contacts because the oral polio vaccine (DPV) may have possible side effects. OPV vaccine is still the vaccine of choice if there should be an outbreak of polio.

Speak with your pediatrician or family physician about the advantages and disadvantages of each vaccine.

The goal to eliminate MEASLES (Rubeola) has unfortunately, not been realized. As a matter-of-fact, there has been reported outbreaks of measles particularly in preschool children, during the last few years. The major cause of these recent outbreaks has been the failure to vaccinate preschool children or failure of the early measles vaccine to be effective. There is reason to believe a possibility exists that persons receiving the measles vaccine prior to 1980 have an increased rate of primary vaccine failure. In mid-1989, an increased number of measles cases was reported in the country, as a result, a major change was made in recommendations for routine immunization for measles. It is now recommended that measles vaccine be given routinely in a 2 dose schedule. The first dose, as before is given at 15 months of age; the second is given upon entry into kindergarten or to middle or junior high school (ask your own doctor to recommend which time).

THE IMPORTANCE OF IMMUNIZATION

In areas where there has been a recent, or is a current outbreak of measles, the American Academy of Pediatrics and Immunization Practices Advisory Committee have recommended the initial measles vaccine be given earlier than 15 months with a further dose at 15 months. Discuss this with your doctor if you live in a community experiencing an outbreak of measles. This is very important because though measles was once thought to be a mild children's disease, it is now known to have possible serious complications such as pneumonia, encephalitis or otitis media (middle ear infection).

RUBELLA. A vaccine is now available for general use against Rubella, some times called German or Three Day Measles. The seriousness of this is greatest for pregnant women. Those who contract the disease in the first three months of pregnancy may have defective or infected babies. Rubella vaccine may be given at 15 months as Measles-Rubella or Measles-Mumps-Rubella combined vaccines.

RESPIRATORY vaccines are still at a developmental stage. In spite of research on the subject, we still have to "sit out" the common cold. One reason is that it may be caused by any of a number of viruses. However, research *has* successfully led to bacterial pneumonia vaccines for "high-risk" children and adults.

Since 1971, the United States Public Health Service has recommended that the routine vaccination against smallpox be discontinued in the United States because risk of the disease is insufficient to justify routine vaccination of infants and children. Smallpox vaccination has occasionally resulted in severe adverse reactions.

HAEMOPHILUS INFLUENZA TYPE B (HIB) disease can now be prevented with a vaccine. HIB bacteria can cause a variety of serious infections, the most dangerous of which are meningitis (inflammation of the membranes covering the brain and spinal cord) and epiglottitis (inflammation of the cartilage at the back of the throat that closes over the airway during swallowing). All children under the age of six risk contracting HIB disease and developing serious after-effects unless vaccinated.

Recently two new vaccines to protect against Haemophilus influenza type B (HIB) has ben approved for use:

One new HIB vaccine is called PRP-T. The other new immunization is a combination vaccine called HbOC-DPT (brand name TETRAMUNE). This vaccine combines protection against diphtheria, tetanus, pertussis (whooping cough) and Haemophilus influenzae type B infections. Combining vaccines should make it easier for more children to be protected. This vaccine is now available for use in infants as young as 2 months of age.

The new schedule will not require additional immunizations.

Your pediatrician or family physician will recommend the schedule for your baby.

HEPATITIS B VACCINE (HBV) The American Academy of Pediatrics (AAP) now recommends all infants be immunized for Hepatitis B. The first dose should be given to newborns before they are discharged from the hospital.

The schedule recommended by AAP is as follows:

HEPATITIS B VACCINE (HBV)

The American Academy of Pediatrics has made the following recommendations:
Recommended Routine Hepatitis B Immunization Schedules

Infant born to Hepatitis B Negative Mothers*

Dose	Age
1	0-2 days
2	1-2 months
3	6-18 month

Infants born to Hepatitis B Positive Mothers**

Dose	Age
1	0 days
2	1 month
3	6 months

*Alternative schedule: dose 1 at 1-2 months of age, dose 2 at 4 months and dose 3 at 6-18 months.

**HBIG also be administered.

For premature and other infants with illnesses in the first few days of life, HBV vaccine may be delayed until hospital discharge "provided" the mother is not HBAg positive.

Hepatitis B Virus vaccine can be given with DTP, Haemophilus influenzae type B, polio, and/or MMR vaccines.

HEALTH RULES

Follow these five simple rules to help your baby stay healthy:
1. Visit your physician or clinic for periodic chechups. Only expert supervision can provide proper and specific protection agaist disease.
2. Teach chilren to wash their hands after using the toilet and before meals.
3. Be sure that the water your children drink and the foods they eat are safe.
4. Cooperate with your local, state and school health programs/agencies.
5. Keep records of all your child's immunizations. In the front of this book you will find a complete chart which can be cut out for your convenience.

Recommended Childhood Immunization Schedule
United States, January - December 1998

Vaccines[1] are listed under the routinely recommended ages. **Bars** indicate range of acceptable ages for immunization. Catch-up immunization should be done during any visit when feasible. Shaded **ovals** indicate vaccines to be assessed and given if necessary during the early adolescent visit.

Age ► Vaccine ▼	Birth	1 mo	2 mos	4 mos	6 mos	12 mos	15 mos	18 mos	4-6 yrs	11-12 yrs	14-16 yrs
Hepatitis B[2,3]	Hep B-1	Hep B-2			Hep B-3					Hep B[3]	
Diphtheria, Tetanus, Pertussis[4]			DTaP or DTP	DTaP or DTP	DTaP or DTP		DTaP or DTP[4]		DTaP or DTP	Td	Td
H influenzae type b[5]			Hib	Hib	Hib	Hib					
Polio[6]			Polio[6]	Polio	Polio	Polio			Polio		
Measles, Mumps, Rubella[7]						MMR			MMR[7]	MMR[7]	
Varicella[8]						VAR	VAR			VAR[8]	

Approved by the Advisory Committee on Immunization Practices (ACIP), the American Academy of Pediatrics (AAP), and the American Academy of Family Physicians (AAFP).

[1]This schedule indicates the recommended age for routine administration of currently licensed childhood vaccines. Some combination vaccines are available and may be used whenever administration of any components of the vaccine is indicated, and are not contraindicated. Providers should consult the manufacturers' package inserts for detailed recommendations.

[2]**Infants born to HBsAg-negative mothers** should receive 2.5 µg of Merck vaccine (Recombivax HB) or 10 µg of SmithKline Beecham (SB) vaccine (Engerix-B). The 2nd dose should be administered at least at 1-2 months of age, and the 3rd dose at 6 months of age.
Infants born to HBsAg-positive mothers should receive 0.5 mL of hepatitis B immune globulin (HBIG) within 12 hrs of birth, and either 5 µg of Merck vaccine (Recombivax HB) or 10 µg of SB vaccine (Engerix-B) at a separate site. The 2nd dose is recommended at 1-2 mos of age and the 3rd dose at 6 mos of age.
Infants born to mothers whose HBsAg status is unknown should receive either 5 µg of Merck vaccine (Recombivax HB) or 10 µg of SB vaccine (Engerix-B) within 12 hrs of birth. The 2nd dose of vaccine is recommended at 1 mo of age and the 3rd dose at 6 mos of age. Blood should be drawn at the time of delivery to determine the mother's HBsAg status; if it is positive, the infant should receive HBIG as soon as possible (no later than 1 wk of age). The dosage and timing of subsequent vaccine doses should be based upon the mother's HBsAg status.

[3]Children and adolescents who have not been vaccinated against hepatitis B in infancy may begin the series during any visit. Those who have not previously received 3 doses of hepatitis B vaccine should initiate or complete the series during the 11 to 12-year-old visit, and unvaccinated older adolescents should be vaccinated whenever possible. The 2nd dose should be administered at least 1 mo after the 1st dose, and the 3rd dose should be administered at least 4 mos after the 1st dose and at least 2 mos after the 2nd dose.

[4]DTap (diphtheria and tetanus toxoids and acellular pertussis vaccine) is the preferred vaccine for all doses in the vaccination series, including completion of the series in children who have received 1 or more doses of whole-cell DTP vaccine. Whole-cell DTP is an acceptable alternative to DTaP. The 4th dose (DTP or DTaP) may be administered as early as 12 months of age, provided 6 months have elapsed since the 3rd dose, and if the child is unlikely to return at 15-18 mos. Td (tetanus and diphtheria toxoids) is recommended at 11-12 years of age if at least 5 years have elapsed since the last dose of DTP, DTaP or DT. Subsequent routine Td boosters are recommended every 10 years.

[5]Three H influenzae type b (Hib) conjugate vaccines are licensed for infant use. If PRP-OMP (PedvaxHIB [Merck]) is administered at 2 and 4 mos of age, a dose at 6 mos is not required.

[6]Two poliovirus vaccines are currently licensed in the US: inactivated poliovirus vaccine (IPV) and oral poliovirus vaccine (OPV). The following schedules are all acceptable to the ACIP, the AAP, and the AAFP. Parents and providers may choose among these options:
     1) 2 doses of IPV followed by 2 doses of OPV.
     2) 4 doses of IPV.
     3) 4 doses of OPV.
The ACIP recommends 2 doses of IPV at 2 and 4 mos of age followed by 2 doses of OPv at 12-18 mos and 4-6 years of age. IPV is the only poliovirus vaccine recommended for immunocompromised persons and their household contacts.

[7]The 2nd dose of MMR is recommended routinely at 4-6 yrs of age but may be administered during any visit, provided at least 1 mo has elapsed since receipt of the 1st dose and that both doses are administered beginning at or after 12 mos of age. Those who have not previously received the second dose should complete the schedule no later than the 11 to 12-year visit.

[8]Susceptible children may receive varicella vaccine (Var) at any visit after the first birthday, and those who lack a reliable history of chickenpox should be immunized during the 11 to 12-year of visit. Susceptible children 13 years of age or older should receive 2 doses, at least 1 month apart.

THE IMPORTANCE OF IMMUNIZATION

COMMUNICABLE DISEASES OF CHILDHOOD*

	Chickenpox	Diphtheria
Cause	A virus: Present in secretions from nose, throat and mouth of infected people.	Diphtheria bacillus: Present in secretions from nose and throat of infected people and carriers.
How Spread	Contact with infected people or articles used by them. Very contagious.	Contact with infected people and carriers or articles used by them.
Incubation period (from date of exposure to first signs)	13 to 17 days. Sometimes 3 weeks.	2 to 5 days. Sometimes longer.
Period of communicability (time when disease is contagious)	From 5 days before to 6 days after first appearance of skin blisters.	From about 2 to 4 weeks after onset of disease.
Most susceptible ages	Under 15 years.	Under 15 years.
Seasons of prevalence	Winter.	Fall, winter and spring.
Prevention	Chickenpox vaccine	Vaccination with diphtheria toxoid (in triple vaccine for babies).
Control	Isolation for 1 week after eruption appears. Avoid contact with susceptibles. Immune globulin may lessen severity. (Cut child's fingernails.) Immunity usual after one attack.	Antitoxin and antibiotics used in treatment and for protection after exposure. One attack does not necessarily give immunity.

*Based on The Control of Communicable Diseases, American Public Health Association, 1982, and Report of Committee on Control of Infectious Diseases, American Academy of Pediatrics, 1982.

THE IMPORTANCE OF IMMUNIZATION

Measles	Mumps	Polio
A virus: Present in secretions from nose and throat of infected people.	A virus: Present in saliva of infected people.	3 strains of polio virus have been identified: Present in discharges from nose, throat, bowels of infected people.
Contact with infected people or articles used by them. Very contagious.	Contact with infected people or articles used by them.	Primarily, contact with infected people.
About 10 to 12 days.	12 to 26 (commonly 18) days.	Usually 7 to 12 days.
From 4 days before until about 5 days after rash appears.	From about 6 days before symptoms to 9 days after. Principally at about time swelling starts.	Apparently greatest in late incubation and first few days of illness.
Common at any age during childhood.	Children and young people.	Most common in children 1 to 16 years.
Mainly spring. Also fall and winter.	Winter and spring.	June through September.
Measles vaccine.	Mumps vaccine.	Polio vaccine.
Isolation until 7 days after appearance of rash. Immune globulin between 3 and 6 days after exposure can lighten attack. Antibiotics for complications. Immunity usual after one attack.	Isolation for 9 days from onset of swelling. Immunity usual after one attack but second attacks can occur.	Isolation for about one week from onset. Immunity to infecting strain of virus usual after one attack.

THE IMPORTANCE OF IMMUNIZATION

	Rheumatic Fever	Rubella
Cause	Direct cause unknown. Precipitated by a strep infection.	A virus: Present in secretions from nose and mouth of infected people.
How spread	Unknown. But the preceding strep infection is contagious.	Contact with infected people or articles used by them. Very contagious.
Incubation period (from date of exposure to first signs)	Symptoms appear about 2 to 3 weeks after a strep infection.	14 to 21 days (usually 18) days.
Period of communicability (time when disease is dangerous)	Not communicable. Preceding strep infection is communicable.	From 7 days before to 5 days after onset of rash.
Most susceptible ages	All ages; most common from 6 to 12 years.	Young children, but also common in young adults.
Seasons of prevalence	Mainly winter and spring.	Winter and spring.
Prevention	No prevention, except proper treatment of strep infections. (See strep infections.)	Rubella (German measles) vaccine.
Control	Use of antibiotics. One attack does not give immunity.	Isolation when necessary, for 5 days after onset. Immunity usual after one attack.

THE IMPORTANCE OF IMMUNIZATION

Strep Infections	Tetanus	Whooping Cough
Streptococci of several strains cause scarlet fever and strep sore throats: Present in secretions from mouth, nose and ears of infected people.	Tetanus bacillus: Present in a wound so infected.	Pertussis bacillius: Present in secretions from mouth and nose of infected people.
Contact with infected people; rarely from contaminated articles.	Through soil, contact with horses, street dust, or articles contaminated with the bacillus.	Contact with infected people and articles used by them.
1 to 3 days.	4 days to 3 weeks. Sometimes longer. Average about 10 days.	From 7 to 10 days.
Greatest during acute illness (about 10 days).	Not communicable from person to person.	From onset of first symptoms to about 3rd week of the disease.
All ages.	All ages.	Under 7 years.
Late winter and spring.	All seasons, but more common in warm weather.	Late winter and early spring.
No prevention. Antibiotic treatment for those who have had rheumatic fever.	Immunization with tetanus toxoid (in triple vaccine for babies).	Immunization with whooping cough vaccine (in triple vaccine for babies).
Isolation for about 1 day after start of treatment with antibiotics — used for about 10 days. One attack does not necessarily give immunity.	Booster dose of tetanus toxoid for protection given on day of injury. Antitoxin used in treatment and for temporary protection for child not immunized. One attack does not give immunity.	Booster doses. Special antibiotics may help to lighten attack for child not immunized. Isolation from susceptible infants for about 3 weeks from onset or until cough stops. Immunity usual after one attack.

CHAPTER 13

Problems and Complaints of Infancy

PARENTS ARE GREAT WORRIERS. Some worry far too much, work themselves into a state of near panic and lose all sense of proportion over every little upset their child may have. The torture of being in such a state of mind is known to all parents. A great flood of relief comes when they finally consult the doctor and find that their fear is unfounded. Some "friend" is always ready to tell a concerned parent about similar cases that turned out badly. A very great deal of their worrying is done unnecessarily because of misinformation. Reading the following may help mothers and fathers worry less.

MINOR ILLNESSES

One reassuring fact is that in infancy major diseases are relatively uncommon. However, at some time or other, you will face different kinds of minor ailments. It will be useful for you to become familiar with some of these. Thus you may be prepared in handling and possibly preventing some of them.

THRUSH may appear in a young baby's mouth as white spots on tongue, cheeks or inside lips. This is distinguished from milk in the mouth because the white spots do not wipe off so readily. It also may have an endocrine relationship. Your doctor will advise you on treatment. You can help to prevent it by more thorough scrubbing of bottles and nipples, turning the latter inside out and scrubbing after each use. Boiling the nipples for a few minutes is advisable. Thrush also appears in some cases after long-term antibiotic therapy.

A SUCKLING BLISTER may appear on a young baby's upper lip. It is caused by frequent and prolonged sucking and has no medical significance.

TEARING OF THE EYES often occurs because of the tear duct opening. This normally drains eye secretions into the nostrils. If it becomes clogged, the secretion is likely to be more or less purulent (containing pus). It appears as if baby has a "cold in the eye." The secretions can be gently wiped off the outside of the eye with a damp cloth. The blockage may only be temporary. But it is one of the things which the doctor will check. Do *not* use boric acid. Don't even have it around the house (see under Poisons).

HERNIA. A hernia is an abnormal opening in the muscle wall which allows some internal organ or organs to protrude. The most common hernia is the umbilical (navel) hernia of the newborn. The actual opening in the navel may be small, big enough only to admit a finger tip, but looks much larger when a bit of intestine or *omentum* (fatty tissue) protrudes through it. This looks alarming. It swells up when the baby strains or cries. But no harm results. By far the greater majority of these will close, including some of the big ones. No treatment is necessary. Rarely does a baby have discomfort from such hernia. If your doctor feels any taping is indicated he will do it.

INGUINAL HERNIA. These are much less common than umbilical hernias and may need surgical repair. Before the modern days of expert surgery on small babies, various kinds of trusses were used. They are all outmoded now. The abnormal opening is around the inguinal region (groin). It allows a bit of intestine to slide back and forth into the scrotum of a boy. This has to be differentiated, by your doctor, from a condition called hydrocele, which is an accumulation of fluid in the scrotum. The two conditions may be associated. In a girl the abnormal swelling will be seen in the groin. Any swelling in these regions should be reported to your doctor. Only rarely, however, is there any emergency associated with it. Your doctor will explain the situation to you.

PERSISTENT SPITTING UP OR VOMITING. Spitting up of milk is most frequently caused by an air bubble in the stomach. It gets underneath the milk and pushes the milk up ahead of it in the "burping" process. When baby is fed sitting upright, the air comes up easily. When he lies down, the air gets underneath the milk. To prevent this type of spitting up, the baby may need to be held in a higher sitting position when fed, and to be "burped" more frequently. A baby who is "hard to burp" may well be fed in an infant seat.

Some babies have a weaker opening into the stomach, causing milk to be regurgitated more frequently. In these babies, the sitting position is all the more important and should be maintained after feeding by propping him up. A helpful system is to raise the head of his mattress by placing a roll under it, such as a rolled up blanket. Do not use a pillow directly under the baby for fear of suffocation.

Should your baby develop "projectile" vomiting - that is vomiting with great force, report this to your doctor immediately.

BOWEL MOVEMENTS IN THE EARLY WEEKS. The stools of a newborn are nothing like the normal stools of childhood. At first they contain a sticky greenish-black secretion, the *meconium*. For several weeks the stool is in a transition between this and the pasty - well-formed stool which comes later. The bowel movement may not assume this latter form until the baby is several months old. Parents need to be reminded at this stage that the appearance of the stools is of much less importance than the thriving condition of the baby. The stools of the breast-fed baby are normally of a scrambled semi-liquid consistency.

MINOR DIARRHEA may occur, often for no obvious reason. The occurrence of some frequency or looseness of stools is not of itself a cause for worry in an otherwise flourishing baby. Laxatives taken by a nursing mother may cause loose stools in her baby. Fruit juices should be omitted during a bout of minor diarrhea.

True CONSTIPATIONS seldom occurs in babies. Infrequency of stools does not necessarily mean the baby is constipated. There will be fewer and scantier stools during an illness when the child is not eating much.

Undue firmness of the stool making it difficult to pass is best regulated by changes in feeding and fluid intake. Prune juice is a more logical laxative than a dose of medicine.

DEHYDRATION

Children under the age of 3 years old need large amounts of fluid. When too much fluid is lost due to diarrhea, vomiting, sweating - symptoms that frequently accompany a fever, dehydration can develop very quickly - if dehydration is prolonged it can be life-threatening.

Newborns and infants with diarrhea and/or vomiting can become dehydrated very rapidly, it is therefore essential that a doctor be consulted immediately. If your doctor can't be reached, take your child to an emergency room immediately.

CONVULSIONS

Convulsions in a child of any age can be very upsetting to a parent. Typical symptoms of a convulsion are (1) stiffening of the body followed by (2) jerky, flailing movements (3) drooling and (4) unconsciousness.

Convulsions can be caused by a high fever, head injury, epilepsy, and infection causing an inflammation of the brain or membrane covering the brain, or even as a result of an allergic reaction.

If your baby (or a child of any age) is having a convulsion it is very important to clear the area nearby of any objects including toys. Do not interfere with child's movements. Do not try to hold child or force anything, including liquids into his mouth.

If the convulsion lasts more than 10 minutes (very rare) call emergency assistance.

Typically it will end sooner, allow child to rest or sleep following the convulsion. Then call your doctor and report symptoms.

TEETHING

Teething seldom causes any real trouble for the baby. But it tends to get blamed for many things. His very first tooth or teeth will most likely come through when baby is between six to eight months old. A baby is getting teeth most of the time between six months and two years. It is only natural to blame teething for upsets that are merely coincidental.

There is no relationship between teething and the rest of the baby's development. There are early-teethers and late teethers. One even hears of a rare baby born with teeth. These are really a third set. They are one or two in number and tend to fall out early. On the other hand, it is not too unusual for teething to start late in the first year. This is no cause for concern.

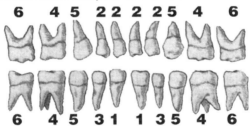

6   4 5   2 2 2 2 5   4   6

6   4 5   3 1   1 3 5   4   6

The order of eruption of teeth can vary too. Again, it means nothing if they are out of the usual sequence. The usual order is as follows:

The 1's tend to erupt together, then the 2's and so on with an interval between the groups.

Sometimes a white spot or "epithelial pearl" appears in the gums prior to teething. It is of no significance except that it may be mistaken for a tooth.

Excessive drooling does accompany teething. Since it may also begin long beforehand, it is not a sign that teething is imminent.

Many parents will say their babies have signs of cold or loose bowel movements when teething. These symptoms may be due to an increase of saliva and mucus.

There may be some fussiness and wakefulness on the part of the baby who is teething, possibly more so when the bigger teeth push through the gums. There may also be a little runny nose and looseness of the bowels. Seldom seen nowadays, however, are the very red, swollen and painful gums that used to require lancing.

If such symptoms do occur, so-called teething lotions are not much help. A little powdered acetaminophen mixed with syrup and applied to the sore gum with your finger will do more good locally. Acetaminophen may also be given by mouth. The proper dose given internally is about one grain per year of age per dose. This should not be given more often than every four hours. If you apply some to the gum, be sure to count it in your dosage for it will, of course, be swallowed and act internally as well. Always observe safety precautions when you are handling medication (See Poisons, page 113.)

Teething almost never causes fever, certainly not high fevers. If fever is present, always suspect illness rather than blame it on teething.

It does seem to give a teething baby relief to bite on something firm, such as a rattle of hard rubber or firm plastic. The leather in his own shoe seems to be just right for this kind of exercise. Teething biscuits are helpful and easy for a baby to hold. The type of teething ring containing fluid which is chilled in the refrigerator does not seem to give enough relief to be worth the bother.

POSSIBLE EFFECTS OF THUMB-SUCKING. Whether prolonged sucking deforms the teeth and jaw has been argued both ways for many years. Cases are seen of prolonged finger-sucking that has definitely caused one-sided deformity of the upper jaw. In this type of finger-sucking, the finger or fingers are turned outward and this exerts great pressure. A thumb may cause deformity of the teeth and jaw in the upper mid-line if pressure is strong enough in a forward direction. Now orthodontists tell us and can demonstrate with models that even the tongue if habitually pressed forward hard enough will deform as much as thumb-sucking. Tongue-sucking can become a habit, too, though a less noticeable one than thumb or

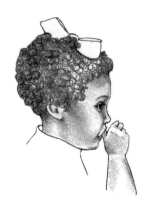

finger-sucking. By and large, however, the average amount of sucking does not deform.

The structure of a baby's teeth can be definitely affected while they are being formed. The first set of teeth begins to form during pregnancy, seven months before birth. They are influenced by the mother's diet, illness and some drugs. The permanent or second set of teeth are laid down during infancy and can be affected by the same kinds of factors during this period. Decay at the gum line of the temporary teeth means that there was some deficiency during pregnancy. Certain antibiotics, if given for a very prolonged period during pregnancy or early infancy, have been found to stain a baby's teeth.

WHAT ABOUT FLUORIDE? Fluoride is a mineral that is important in formation of sound teeth and their preservation from decay. Surveys have shown that there is less tooth decay in communities which have added fluoride to the water supply. The safety of fluoride has been thoroughly checked by leading public health and dental authorities. Where fluoride has been kept out of the water supply because of misguided opposition, it can be obtained by prescription from the doctor either as such or combined with vitamins. With the latter you are less likely to forget to administer it.

MINOR SKIN RASHES

"My baby has a rash!" is probably one of the most common complaints the baby's doctor hears. Some of these rashes are defined for you in the chart at the bottom of this page. In most instances you will not be satisfied until the doctor sees the rash, gives it a name and advises you on what to do or not do.

HEAT RASH or "PRICKLY HEAT" occurs in hot weather in babies who are overdressed. A young baby's sweat glands are rather sluggish. They do not function efficiently, if at all, when the baby is wrapped too warmly.

SEBORRHEA is a peculiar type of greasy scaling then occurs in some babies. It occurs mostly in eyebrows and scalp where it may be called "cradle cap."

ECZEMA occurs on the face or may be distributed over the body. In most instances it is an allergic condition. It nearly always itches severely.

Other SENSITIVITY RASHES may be due to over-medication. Baby oil is one of the worst offenders. External as well as internal medication may sensitize a baby, as well as an adult.

DIAPER RASHES. This area is the most often irritated by contact with bowel movements (especially if diarrhea) or with urine. Urine itself is not irritating. But the combination of prolonged wetness, warmth and lack of air causes most diaper rashes. Infant boys can get severe irritation of penis and scrotum from sleeping face down with waterproof pants on all night. Treatment consists of exposing the area to air frequently during the day and omitting the plastic pants. Healthy infants should be placed on their backs or sides to sleep.

Another cause of irritation in the diaper area is washing the diapers with detergents that are too strong. The usual washing machine cycle generally does not rinse the diapers thoroughly enough. Diapers could well be run through an extra cycle with plain water.

If your baby does develop a diaper rash, don't wait until it becomes severe to take action. There are steps you can take early-on so the condition does not become worse: (1) Change baby often including at night, even if baby is asleep. (2) Expose baby's bottom to the air as much s possible. If using disposable diapers, change brands; some babies may develop an allergy to one

OTHER SKIN RASHES IN INFANCY

Name	Impetigo	Intertrigo	Sensitivity Dermatitis
Location and appearance	Any skin area; scattered scabs or pustules; spreads on contact.	Body folds, groin, neck, armpits; redness and moisture where skin surfaces rub together.	Mild redness or roughness of face or body.
Cause	Secondary infection getting into break in the skin.	Same combination of causes as diaper rash, plus low grade infection.	Possible sensitivity to orange juice or to baby oil.
Treatment	Antibiotic ointment.	Bland ointment or cornstarch.	Unnecessary.
Prevention	Cleanse cuts and apply antiseptic.	Apply cornstarch after drying.	Use Vitamin C instead of orange juice; use soap and water rather than baby oil.

brand but not another. Avoid using baby wipes that contain alcohol while baby has a rash because it can cause stinging and pain.

Occasionally the sudden onset of a rash can be traced to a new food introduced into baby's diet, particularly foods such as tomatoes and citrus foods which have a high acid content.

COLDS AND COUGHS

COLDS IN YOUNG INFANTS. Colds are not so common in early infancy as later. When a cold does occur, there is more likely to be a general stuffiness of nose than the profuse nasal discharge of an older child. Hence it may not be so obvious that a baby has a cold. Stomach-sleeping is not desirable for a baby with a cold. It may further reduce his breathing space. You will want to check on the baby several times during the night to keep him changed and dry and to see that he is not developing any breathing difficulty. The latter always requires medical care.

There is no treatment which will cure the common cold or shorten it in any way. Antibiotics are ineffective. Some medications will give symptomatic relief for the extremely stuffy nose or excessive mucus or overly troublesome cough. It never does any good to "rub something on the chest." This only irritates the skin. Neither is it good to wrap a child in too many warm garments and blankets in the vain hope of "sweating it out." Where fever is present, over-dressing may aggravate it greatly by sending the temperature much higher.

For a profusely runny nose, one can gently suction out the discharge with a soft rubber bulb syringe. This may give much relief to a child too young to blow his nose. It is better than constant wiping with tissue which makes the nostrils sore.

At one time steam inhalation, using room humidifiers such as vaporizers or cool misters was recommended as the best and most soothing treatment for upper respiratory infections and irritations. It was found, however, that these humidifiers were breeding grounds for disease causing bacteria and fungi (molds), and that these organisms were being spewed into the air by the mist.

In December, 1988, the U.S. Consumer Product Safety Commission (CPSC) issued an "Alert" regarding the newer Ultrasonic humidifiers.

Because the ultrasonic humidifiers use high frequency vibrations which changes water into mist, no live mold and few bacteria were being spread into the air - thus making them safer. However, recent tests have indicated that when tap water is used with these humidifiers (and most people do use tap water to fill their humidifiers even when directions call for distilled water), tiny particles of minerals dissolved in the water, are dispersed by the mist into the air. These minerals form a white dust and when the dust is inhaled, it reaches the deepest parts of the lungs were it can aggravate chronic diseases such as asthma and bronchitis. Tests also indicated this dust may increase a child's susceptibility to upper respiratory infections such as colds and/or flu.

The U.S. Environmental Agency (EPA) also warns of these dangers. Their studies indicated ultrasonic humidifiers, using tap water, filled a test room with mineral particles, forty times the recommended limit for outdoor air.

The EPA therefore recommends - if ultrasonic humidifiers are used - that filters capable of removing minerals from water be added and that only distilled water be used with any humidifier.

Ultrasonic humidifiers - as well as other types of humidifiers - *must* be cleaned daily to prevent bacteria and fungi from growing and being spewed into the air.

Do not use any room humidifier without first discussing this with your doctor, particularly if your child has allergies, asthma, or chronic bronchitis.

CROUP or LARYNGITIS is common in older infants and children. The "cold" in this case is in the child's vocal chords. It causes a hoarse "barking" cough which may recur for several nights. Do not use humidifiers/vaporizers without first checking with your doctor. (See pages 99-100 the EPA and CPSC recommendations on the use of vaporizers/humidifiers.)

EAR INFECTIONS occur in children more often than in adults because of the anatomy of the ear and the Eustachian tube connecting the nose to the middle ear. An ear infection is nearly always a complication of a cold. A draining ear is much more serious than a "runny" nose. It should always have treatment. It is considerably better to get treatment *before* it drains: when a child first complains of an earache, or when his irritability and crying make you suspect that he might have an earache. Call your doctor promptly. Do not put anything in the ear without first consulting with your doctor.

PREVENTION OF COLDS. Colds are caused by viruses. One "catches" them from an infected person. It is advisable to isolate a baby as much as possible when other members of the family have colds.

There is no evidence that chilling causes colds unless the virus is already present. Chilling certainly can make a cold worse. So sensible dress is important, though not over-dressing. Keep the lower part of the baby's body covered, as well as the upper part, to help prevent chilling from drafts on the floor.

Common sense dictates that children with colds should not be allowed out in the cold with bare legs and no underwear or in the rain with no head covering, boots, or rubbers.

COUGHING is a complaint for which parents frequently request medical advise. There are different types of coughs. There are different causes of coughing. And there are may different cough remedies.

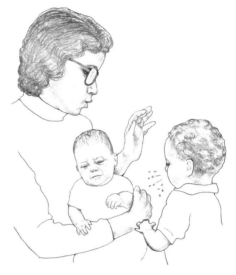

A cough may even be useful, as for example, when it brings up mucus or phlegm that is irritating the throat or lower respiratory tract. This type of cough should not be entirely suppressed by strong cough medication.

A mild cough may require no treatment. Many minor little "hacks" are due to a slight irritation of the throat and are soothed by frequent sips of water. Drink a lot of fluid will also help a "tight" cough by "loosening" thick phlegm.

On the other hand, a child can become worn out with constant coughing. Liquid cough medicines containing expectorants may also be required. An allergic cough will call for a still different prescription. For these complex reasons, cough medicines bought over the drug store counter are less effective than a doctor's prescription.

The best all-around home remedy for most coughs is frequently to give the child liquid to drink. For the more severe coughs, a doctor's prescription is usually necessary.

THE QUESTION OF PETS

The question of the advisability of a pet for a child comes up frequently. A parent will often think it will be so nice to get a puppy or kitty and have it "grow up along with baby." It must be remembered that the animal will grow up much faster and that its life span is much shorter. The child may have to part with it at an age when it may seem very tragic to him. There are many advantages to a child in having a warm relationship with an animal, especially if he can consider it his own. There are many disadvantages, too, particularly with babies and young children.

There are some diseases which a young child can get from pets. The most common is ringworm from puppies or kittens. While the intestinal parasites (worms) of animals are specific for them and not humans, the larvae of one kind can be picked up by children who eat dirt and show up as a peculiar type of skin rash.

There is little danger of rabies or distemper now that dogs have a good immunization program. For safety, however, frequent examination of pets in the first year is as good an idea as it is for babies.

ALLERGY TO PETS. Perhaps the greatest argument against having a cat or dog is the question of allergy in the child. Such pets are high on the list of allergens to which a potentially allergic (that is, with a strong family history of allergy) child can become sensitized. Nor can this possibility be ruled out with skin tests, for it may take as long as two years of continuous exposure for a child to become sensitized. Since desensitization to pets is difficult or next to impossible, avoidance in the first place is the best policy. Then, too, it is much easier to refuse to get the pet at all than it is to get rid of it once it causes trouble.

As for other pets, birds are out for the allergic child. Feathers are frequently more irritating than pet fur. Some birds of the parakeet family may carry parrot fever or psittacosis. Even turtles have been known to carry infections. This leaves goldfish or guppies as possible alternatives but they are not very much fun for a child.

DOG BITES. Children should be trained early to avoid strange animals and never to disturb any dog when it is eating. Be on the alert for dangerous dogs in your area. Keep your child away from yards where such dogs are fenced in. The best first aid treatment for dog bites is to wash the wound with soap and water. Telephone your doctor for additional advice.

REYE'S SYNDROME AND THE USE OF ASPIRIN

Ordinarily, aspirin is a wonder drug, but in 1982 the FDA proposed that it should *not* be given for influenza, chicken pox or other flu-like illnesses. The recommendation comes after the discovery of circumstantial links between aspirin and Reye's Syndrome.

Reye's Syndrome is an acute condition which may develop following influenza (flu), chicken pox or other viral infections which cause flu-like symptoms. It can occur from infancy on through the teen years. The symptoms are sudden vomiting, severe headaches and changes in behavior. This condition requires immediate diagnosis and admission to a hospital where emergency care can be provided. Reye's Syndrome is rare but when it does occurs it is considered life-threatening.

Reye's occurs most frequently from October to March, during the so called "flu season," and seems to be most prevalent in those states reporting the cases of influenza.

Studies have shown an association or link between children under the age of 16 taking aspirin for flu-like symptoms and viral illnesses and developing Reye's Syndrome. Therefore "the Food and Drug Aministration (FDA) has proposed that aspirin and other salicylates and medication containing aspirin, be labled with a *warning* against giving them to children under the age of 16 with influenza, chicken pox or other flu-like illnesses."

The American Academy of Pediatrics recommends not using aspirin or products containing aspirin if your child has a fever. As a matter of fact, many doctors advise against the use of aspirin in children in any situation.

Instead, acetaminophen can be used to reduce fever or relieve pain. Follow directions on the label unless otherwise recommended by your doctor.

Acetaminophen is the active ingredient in Tylenol, Anacin 3 and Panadol to name a few. All are available in children's chewable tablets and liquid drops for infants. Check with your doctor as to which one he/she recommends.

It is essential to read labels on medications carefully - many over-the-counter medications contain aspirin even though the brand name doesn't indicate this.

Reye's Syndrome, according to the U.S. Department of Health is always a medical emergency and must be treated in a hospital.

CHAPTER 14

Accidents

THANKS TO MODERN ADVANCES in public health and preventive medicine, your child is less likely to have a serious disease than you were in your infancy. When and if he does become ill, his doctor has improved diagnostic tools and immeasurably greater resources for his treatment than was available a generation ago.

No such advances have been made in preventing a child from having accidents. According to the National Safety Council, accidents kill more children than all childhood diseases combined. Their toll in disability and suffering is incalculable.

Since so many of these tragedies take place in the home, we must conclude that the average American household, even with its high standard of living, is not geared to raising children nor made safe for them. Indeed the very abundance of new products for the maintenance of a complex household exposes the child to often-unrecognized poisons. New "extra strength" products stridently compete on TV for you to buy them. Some are also "extra poisonous."

If as many accidents happened in an industrial plant as do in the home, the managers would quickly make a survey. On the basis of their findings, they would install guards and make safety regulations. Such studies have been made in analyzing home accidents. These are some of the things they show:

Most childhood accidents happen in the early morning before the parents are up and in the late afternoon when mother is busy getting dinner. In other words, when parental supervision is lax or entirely lacking.

Some parts of the house have been found to be more hazardous than others. In the average home, most accidents occur in the kitchen, the bathroom next, then bedroom and basement. The garage is a bad place to play if pesticides, garden sprays, paint and kerosene products are stored there.

Even the garden may have its hazards with poisonous plants, both cultivated and wild. You should not be denied a beautiful garden. But you should be aware that some plants, with berries and seeds that are likely to attract a child, are deadly. These vary in different regions so you need to seek local information. This is readily available from Poison Control Centers.

ACCIDENTS

All this sounds very fearsome, as indeed it is, but you can do a great deal to protect your children by anticipating some of the explorations and experiments that they are likely to make and by rearranging your house and yard accordingly. Your objective will be to have a safe house rather than a pretty one, at least during the pre-school years of the child. This is when he is the most accident-prone because of the very nature of his growth and development: his urge to explore and to try everything and his tendency to put *everything in his mouth*.

POSSIBLE HAZARDS - BY ROOM

KITCHEN - the most dangerous room (not a good place to play)
because of:

- Hot stoves and oven doors.
- Hot iron, with dangling cord. Hot plate.
- Pans on stove. Always turn handles inward.
- Gas jets which might get turned on, or leak.
- Matches. Keep them out of sight.
- Electric mixer or blender in operation.
- Spilled grease or liquids on floor.
- Broken glass. It should be mopped up with a damp paper towel.
- Foods which can cause choking: nuts (peanuts are most frequent), popcorn, dried peas or beans, small candies.
- Cleaning liquids and powders. Keep locked in cupboard even though inconvenient. Especially beware of:

     Dishwasher detergent (electrical type)
     Drain cleaner (do not keep this at all)
     Bleaches
     Household ammonia
     Dry cleaning fluids
     Spot cleaners
     Furniture and metal polish.
- High-chair. Never leave child alone in high chair. Put him down before you answer the phone or the doorbell.
- Use no tablecloths.
- Hot coffee or soup should never be within child's sudden reach.
- Unlabeled bottles. Leave things in original containers.

BATHROOM - the second most dangerous room.

- All medicines should be locked up as soon as used.

ACCIDENTS

- Read labels before using.
- Never take or give medicine in the dark.
- Cosmetics, hair preparations, powders and depilatories should also be locked up.
- Talcum powder is no longer recommended for infants. It can be irritating to the skin and mucous membrane making it particularly dangerous when it is inhaled. Cornstarch can be used instead of talcum if baby has diaper rash or irritation.
- Avoid slippery floors. Wipe up water and try to teach "no running" in the bathroom.
- Keep razor blades locked up.
- Put safety pins in soap or pin cushion out of reach.
- If you must leave the room for any reason, wrap baby in towel and take baby with you.
- Fix door lock or leave it off so child cannot lock himself in.
- Never leave a child alone in bathtub, even for one second.
  Have all supplies ready and within reach before putting baby in tub.
- Never leave water standing in the tub.
- Use no electrical appliances which may fall in the water, such as razor or radio.
- Permanent wave solutions strong enough to curl your hair will do worse than "curl" in a stomach.

BEDROOM AND SEWING ROOM - third most dangerous room.

- Tippy bureau or chest might be climbed on (and often is).
- Powder and perfume should be put away.
- Moth balls are poisonous, especially naphthalene type or camphor.
- Small objects - jewelry, buttons, coins, thimbles can cause trouble if put in mouth. Sharp objects - pins, needles, cuticle scissors are also dangerous.
- Suggestions when sewing - keep scissors in cork, thimble over it.

LIVING ROOM

- Fireplace. Keep screened at all times. Beware of loose, inflammable clothing, especially nightgowns too close to fireplace.
- Fireplace crystals are poisonous if swallowed.
- Cigarette lighters, because of poisonous fluid or flame.
- Cigarette butts and match heads should be thrown out promptly.
- Frayed electric cords will give shock in a wet mouth.
- Cords by which child might pull down lamp or telephone on himself.

ACCIDENTS

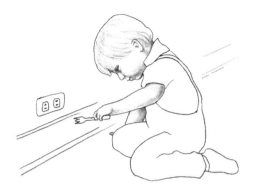

BUY PLASTIC GUARDS FOR SOCKETS

- Electric outlets and sockets. Get plastic guards.
- Tippy floor lamps.
- Glass ornaments or glass edge of coffee table.
- Glass doors. Make visible by gluing decorations at child's level.
- Windows should be well screened.
- Dangerous playthings - coins, buttons, needles, pins, eyes and squeakers from toys.
- Hot pipes and radiators. Registers can cause "waffle" pattern burn.
- House plants, such as "Dumb Cane" (Dieffenbachia), if chewed.

NURSERY

- Crib bars should not be more than two and three-eights inches apart.
- Use non-toxic indoor paint if repainting an old crib.
- Never leave crib sides down.
- Use no harness or zipper bag. Do not tie baby to crib in any way.
- No toy or removable part of toy should be smaller than baby's mouth.
- Animal eyes or squeaker may fall out or get pulled off.
- Sharp or broken toys may be fallen on.
- Leave no venetian blind cords near crib.
- There should be a firm mattress. No pillow or soft pads.
- Beware of plastic bags in crib or near baby.
- Keep crib away from windows. Once baby can stand up in his crib and bounce up and down, a near-by window is a danger.

ACCIDENTS

STAIRS
- Keep well lighted, with banister.
- Use gate at top and bottom of stairwell.
- Have fire extinguishers readily available.
- Keep basement door closed with firm spring or high hook.
- Walk upstairs behind and downstairs in front of a child who is just learning to walk up and down or fence off steps.

GARAGE AND BASEMENT (Best to keep door locked and child out)
- Sharp tools, power tools, mowers, nails, tacks, screws, rusty nails.
- Poisons: insecticides, pesticides - rat and ant poisons are especially bad.
- Garden sprays, weed killer, DDT.
- Kerosene or gasoline.
- Paint products.
- Stored plant bulbs. Some are poisonous when eaten.

YARD AND GARDEN, NEIGHBORHOOD.
- Use gates, fence without sharp pickets, porch railing.
- Pick up broken glass, tin cans.
- Wading pools, fish ponds and even puddles need constant supervision.
- Poisonous plants: a surprising number, both cultivated and wild, are poisonous. Garden examples: Laburnum, the yellow golden chain has clusters of sweet pea-like flowers which become pods, containing very poisonous seeds. Red berries of Daphne mezereum, Skimmia japonica plant. Wild plants: Green berries of False Nightshade, Yew needles, Poison Hemlock, a weed with purple splotches on the stems.
- Find out about the poison plants in your area.
- Teach child very early never to put any plant material in his mouth.

CAR ACCIDENTS
- Children are safer in cars when they ride in the rear seat and have some type of seat restraint. Groups which have studied crash injury accidents advise the following rules for the protection of children
  Infants: Car carrier facing rear.
  Toddlers: Strong child carrier secured by seat belt.
  Older Child: Standard lap seat belt. May sit on a cushion to increase field of vision.
- Children should not ride unrestrained in open areas, such as rear of station wagons, trucks, rear shelf of passenger cars, playpens or as standees.
- All doors should be locked from the inside when vehicle is in motion.

- Do not place objects on the rear shelf. These can become missiles in a sudden stop.
- Check tires for possible defects and proper inflation. Avoid overloading.

CAR AND DRIVEWAY

- Driveways are dangerous where car backs out. Tricycles are often involved in this type of accident, being below range of driver's vision.
- Fence off driveway. Keep child from playing in driveway.
- Use recommended infant car carrier in the back seat.
- Do not buy child's car seat which has attached toy steering wheel.
- Keep car doors locked when under way.
- Never leave child alone in car.

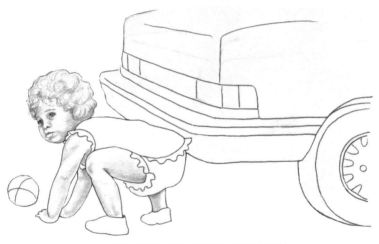

KEEP BABY OUT OF THE DRIVEWAY

BURNS

Most burn accidents are needless tragedies. Many happen to toddlers who fall on hot heat registers or make sudden grabs toward hot liquids placed too near them. An unattended child may turn on hot water when left in a bathtub. Older children play with matches or get too near open heaters or flames when wearing inflammable, loose clothing. A number of children have been burned when their nightgowns caught fire from an open fireplace. Loose fitting clothing should not be worn near the kitchen stove, fireplace or open space heater. Even shirt tails hanging out have led to such accidents. Bedding should not be near heat source. Some types of fabrics and party costumes and even toys have been highly flammable. Some laws governing the flammability of manufactured objects and materials have been passed, but you should always check labels before buying.

Despite the partial ban on fireworks, hundreds of accidents involving them occur each year. Fireworks booths set up at the edge of prohibited areas do a flourishing business. One sees parents lined up here, too, as well as children, willing to buy danger.

Parent supervision is still the most important fire and burn preventive.

DROWNING

As neighborhood swimming pools become more numerous, children will be more exposed to drowning hazards. There may be such dangers even closer to home. A small child can drown in just a few inches of water, in a puddle, fishpond or even the bathtub. Drowning can be instantaneous in a young child. You may not even have time to use mouth to mouth resuscitation. Prevention by supervision and fencing off of pools and puddles is most urgent and necessary.

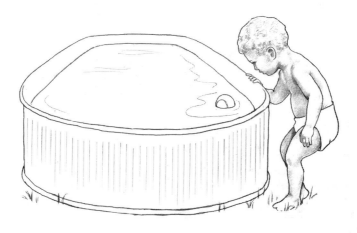

ACCIDENTS

HOW SAFE ARE YOUR CHILD'S TOYS?

Since 1973, the U.S. Consumer Products Safety Commission has taken action in hundreds of cases to stop the sale of unsafe toys and inflammable clothing. Despite their efforts, many toys are still dangerous. Imported toys which are not so regulated may appear on the market before their defects and dangers are discovered. Actual contamination with disease germs was discovered in a teething device containing polluted river water from Hong Kong, and in toy chicks made of real skin and feathers imported from Japan.

A Polish doll was highly inflammable when placed near heat, but broken toys and the misuse of toys are far more common causes of accidents. The trouble then is faulty parental supervision. Sometimes a parent will give a toy to a child who is too young to use it well, such as a wheeled vehicle that may carry him into danger.

BICYCLE-MOUNTED CHILD SEATS

A recent study revealed a "marked increase" in injuries to bicycle passengers under the age of five as well as a concurrent increase in bicycle mounted child seats. Over 65% of these injuries were to the head and face. If you are going to mount a child seat on your bicycle be certain your child is wearing an appropriate helmet whenever riding in this seat.

BABY-SITTERS

In many cities there are club groups which instruct baby-sitters in safety measures. By supporting and participating in these groups you can make sitters more valuable to you. Because they are the parents of tomorrow, they need to be better versed in these matters.

As a conscientious parent, you will not be satisfied merely to read this chapter and check the list for hazards in your home. There are many pamphlets on safety put out by the National Safety Council, the Red Cross, insurance companies, manufacturers of baby food and baby products, the American Medical Association, the Academy of Pediatrics and some local clubs. Read all you can get hold of, especially those booklets that refer to your local area. There are also government bulletins and many magazine articles in the health and home-making field. Promote safety programs as topics for discussion in your PTA and other groups. Safety is one of the major problems in child care today.

SOME REASSURANCE

While it is unlikely that these accidents will happen to you or your family, you should be forewarned of the possibilities. Do not become so fearful that you hover too much over your baby or keep him overly restrained or torture yourself with constant worry. Beware and be aware of the common sources of danger and take preventive action.

CHAPTER 15

Accidental Poisoning

POISONING ACCIDENTS ARE THE most frequent type of mishap involving children. It is estimated that approximately 500,00 cases of childhood poisoning occur in the United States each year. Some 500 of these prove fatal. Many others have serious effects.

The main reason is that almost every child of pre-school age is naturally curious. He will test many things by putting them in his mouth. Even bad taste is often not a deterrent.

Part of the trouble, too, is that we have many products for keeping our houses cleaned, polished and painted which may be poisonous. Drain cleaners, dishwasher detergents, bathroom cleaners, furniture and metal polishes, kerosene products such as lighter fluid, must all be handled with care when in use and kept *locked* away from children when not in use.

Many products will say on the label "Keep out of reach of children." But a busy parent does not always read the fine print.

TV advertising compounds the problem by rarely giving its commercials any warning about potential hazards. "Extra strength" cleaners and medicines may contain ingredients which may well make them "extra poisonous."

But it is probably lack of proper parental supervision which is the biggest cause of poisoning accidents. Experts estimate that if parents would only remember to keep these materials out of sight and reach of children, at least three out of four of these accidents could be prevented.

POISON CONTROL CENTERS

Poison control centers now exist in practically every area. These centers have been of great benefit in saving lives. They also give advice on poisoning and possible poisoning. One example is the Chicago Poison Control Center which takes an average of 14,000 to 15,000 calls involving children up to age two, sends 2,250 of them for outpatient treatment, 500 for extended hospital stays and most years does not have a single death for the age group. This remarkable record is duplicated all over the United States. In addition, such centers have information about the composition of old and new products and their possible effects, whether hazardous or not.

ACCIDENTAL POISONING

Poison Control Centers operate night and day. The telephone number should always be kept handy along with that of your doctor, who should be called first in an emergency. The files at these centers are crammed with case histories of accidents that never should have occurred. (For more information on what to do in case of poisoning, see My Poison Control Guide, p. 132.)

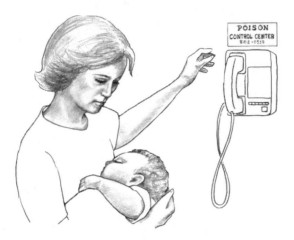

ALWAYS KEEP THE POISON CONTROL CENTER NUMBER HANDY

Here is one example: Tyrone and Maria had been playing in the neighborhood and came home vomiting. They were carrying some sample bottles that they had found on neighborhood doorsteps. These turned out to be promotion "giveaways" of a powerful new household cleanser which had been distributed that morning. The printing on the sample bottles gave no clue as to the ingredients or whether they were poisonous when taken internally. It was too new to be on the list at the local poison control center. A long distance telephone call was placed by the Poison Control Center to the manufacturer's headquarters located far away. Because of the difference in time zones, the office was closed. Alert telephone operators were able to reach the home of the company president. They finally ascertained that the ingredients were not deadly and would have no effects other than the vomiting. With some household substances such a delay, the story might have had a tragic ending.

ACCIDENTAL POISONING

Some household products are so dangerous that you should not keep them around at all. In many cases, they are not that useful or necessary. Drain cleaner, which contains lye, an extremely corrosive substance, is not needed in modern drains. Recently it has been falsely promoted as a disinfectant to "kill the germs in your sink." This is a fallacy since the germs in your sink are not disease-causing. Even if they were, using anything as powerful as lye to kill them would be like using an "elephant gun" for a mouse.

Some dishwasher detergents are also corrosive, though less so than lye. All should be kept locked up when not in use. Although this may be inconvenient, you should either lock the kitchen cupboard doors or find a method of tying them securely shut as a deterrent to a child "on the prowl."

Some furniture and metal polishes may also be injurious. Their fragrant smell often attracts a child to them, while the furniture is being dusted or polished.

Mothballs containing camphor or naphthalene should not be used in a household where there are small children.

THE MEDICINE CHEST

KEEP IT LOCKED AT ALL TIMES! It is not enough to store medicine on a high shelf. A frequent mother's or father's lament at the Poison Control Center is, "But I never knew he could climb so high!"

Jacqueline's parents thought they had done all the "right" things. They purchased baby tylenol with the so called "safety" cap or "childproof" cap on it and placed it up high in a cupboard where they assumed 2 1/2 year old Jacqueline could not climb. But Jackie did climb up. She managed to open the cap and ate three fourths of the bottles contents. Fortunately, this was soon discovered and reported to both the doctor and the Poison Control Center. The doctor advised the parents to get a bottle of Syrup of Ipecac at the drug store and to give Jacqueline one dose to make her vomit. This type of treatment is frequently used. In about fifteen minutes Jackie began to retch. They held her head low over a basin and up came some still recognizable pills.

Medicines accessible to the child cause most of the poisoning trouble. Before the advent of Poison Control Centers, aspirin alone caused the death of about 100 children a year in the United States. Poison Control Centers handle around 100 cases of aspirin poisoning a month. In most instances it is the candy-like flavor of children's medicine that prompts children to eat it. It may even be represented as "candy" to persuade the child to take it for an illness. After much pressure from pediatricians and public health authorities, a law finally has been passed limiting the number of pills to no more than 36 in bottles of baby non-prescription medicine. This is still too much at one dose but at least it is better than the large bottles of regular or extra strength adult pain, allergy or fever medication which unfortunately are not regulated.

Since children keep getting into medicines however, the best idea is to keep on hand only a small amount of the regular size tablets. It is cheap enough. You never really need to buy a big "bargain" bottle.

Prescription drugs taken by adults several times a day are seldom put away. They may be found in bureau drawers or Mommy's purse or on the dining table. Some of the ones most harmful to children in overdose are iron pills, tranquilizers and "reducing" pills. Liniment used for sore joints may have Oil of Wintergreen in it. As little as one teaspoonful may be a fatal dose. If you are sure you really need the liniment, lock it up right after use *without delay*.

There are some outmoded medicines still found in medicine chests. For safety's sake they ought not be there. Boric acid and camphorated oil are examples. The medicine chest needs to be cleared out periodically to get rid of these and other unlabeled medicines. Never keep anything, such as permanent wave liquids, in other than its original container. Cosmetics should also be kept out of reach of children. Chemicals in cosmetics and colognes are toxic when ingested.

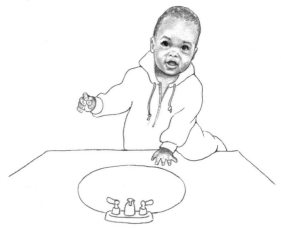

"I DIDN'T KNOW HE COULD REACH!"

ACCIDENTAL POISONING

PRINCIPLES OF POISONING TREATMENT

In the past it was customary to get rid of a poison which had been swallowed by "pumping the stomach." It was not really a pump but rather a rubber tube passed down for washing out the stomach contents. This may still be necessary on occasion. However, the modern method of making the child vomit by giving Syrup of Ipecac is easier and more effective. Some poisons, such as bleaches, will themselves cause vomiting.

Diluting the poison by having the child drink fluids is an important First Aid measure before inducing vomiting. Drinking milk or water may be recommended by your healthcare professional. Liquids in large amount are necessary to dilute the poison.

There are few specific antidotes to the many poisons that exist. In general, you should not spend time looking them up. Occasionally, the label of a package or bottle will give an antidote to the contents, if swallowed. But an immediate call to your doctor and Poison Control Center will get you the best advice.

EXCEPTIONS to the First Aid rule of making a child vomit the poison are few but important. In the case of corrosive poisons (drain cleaner, dishwasher detergents) or kerosene products (kerosene, lighter fluid, turpentine) and some others, vomiting may do more harm than good. This is why you MUST CALL YOUR DOCTOR AND POISON CONTROL CENTER FIRST.

Call 911 promptly if your child has swallowed a toxic substance and exhibits any of the following symptoms:

- Difficulty breathing
- Sudden changes in behavior
- Unexplained nausea vomiting
- Stomach pains without a fever
- Burns on your child's lips or mouth

CHAPTER 16

A Few ABC's on First Aid

IN SPITE OF YOUR best efforts accidents will happen. And you must "cope" with them. A knowledge of some of the updated fundamentals of First Aid will help you.

BURNS

Apply cool water, not grease. Call your doctor. If deep enough to blister, bring child to doctor. If extensive enough to hospitalize, wrap child in damp sheet for transporting. Sunburn: Prevent! Keep child covered with clothing rather than wearing "those darling little sunsuits" that allow burns of shoulders and back.

BLEEDING

If extensive, apply pressure with palm of hand. Do not use a tourniquet, but rather a pressure bandage - layers of folded gauze held in place with tape or by hand.

Gently wash any cut with dirt in it or one that does not bleed freely. Do not use iodine. Mercurochrome may be used if child is not sensitive to it. If cut is gaping, it will probably need suturing (stiches). Small gaping cuts can be pulled together with tape, but may leave scar.

Cut in mouth may be washed with diluted hydrogen peroxide (diluted to half strength with water).

Tetanus toxoid booster is advisable for dirty wounds, especially if any horse manure was nearby.

CHOKING (on object)

If the child is not breathing, turn his head to one side, hold him face down over your knees and thump him vigorously. If the choking child is an infant, place him over your forearm instead.

If a child who is choking on a foreign body is crying, coughing or talking, it is best to allow the child's own reflexes to relieve the obstruction or foreign body. If, however, the baby is not breathing or is unable to make sounds, immediate first aid is essential according to the policy statement issued in the September issue of Pediatrics.

A FEW ABC's ON FIRST AID

The Heimlich maneuver (see Figure 1) is still recommended for children <u>one year</u> of age or older.

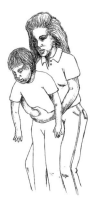

FIGURE 1. Abdominal thrusts with conscious victim standing or sitting (for children 1 year of age or older).

Though there is still some disagreement concerning what first aid management should be taken for the choking child under 12 months of age, the American Academy of Pediatricfs, in its 1993 policy guidelines, recommends 5 back blows (see Figure 2) followed by 5 chest thrusts (see Figure 3).

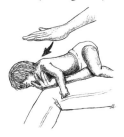
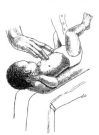

The Heimlich maneuver (abdmominal thrust technique) may injure the internal organs such as the stomach, liver or spleen of children under the age of 12 months.

A FEW ABC's ON FIRST AID

Parents, as well as other family members, should learn how to do these emergency first aid procedures. There are formal training classes sponsored by the American Heart Association and the American Red Cross. Consult with your baby's doctor if you have any questions on first aid for your baby in case of choking. If child is still not breathing, open his mouth, holding the jaw with your finger and placing your thumb on the tongue. If you see something, remove it with your other hand. If none of these measures succeds, rush child to hospital or doctor without delay. Prevent, by not allowing small child any peanuts (or other nuts), popcorn, small candies or tiny toys. Hot dogs and whole grapes are also hazardous.

CONVULSIONS

A convulsion is not always an emergency although it is admittedly frightening. Reduce fever, if present, by sponge bath or damp towel wrapped around child's body. Leave blankets and clothing off. Lower the room temperature if possible.

ANIMAL BITES

Call the doctor as soon as baby's condition has stabilized. Wash well with soap and water. Report bite to local police and health department. Try to keep track of the animal. Teach child not to pet a strange dog or any dog when it is eating.

DROWNING

Get child to a hospital. Have someone call doctor.

Do not take time to drain out the water for it is absorbed immediately through the lungs.

If anything is in the mouth, wipe it out quickly with your fingers or a handkerchief.

Mouth to mouth resuscitation should be given immediately and on the way to the hospital.

TECHNIQUE OF MOUTH TO MOUTH RESUSCITATION
(approved by the American Red Cross).

Place child in face up position. Tilt his head back so the chin points upward. Lift the lower jaw from below so that it juts forward and hold. If necessary, clear the child's mouth and throat of any obstruction.

Place your mouth over the child's mouth and nose, making a leak-proof seal. Breathe into the child's lungs, using very, very shallow puffs of air. Count five between puffs, making a breathing rate of about 20 per minute.

A FEW ABC's ON FIRST AID

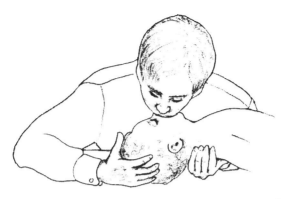

Your mouth over baby's mouth and nose. Tilt his head back and make certain his tongue is not obstructing air passage.

If you meet resistance in your blowing effort, recheck the position of the jaw, pushing it forward. This gets the tongue out of the way. If air passages seem blocked, suspend the child momentarily by the ankles. Give him two or three pats (not blows) between the shoulder blades to dislodge obstructing matter.

FRACTURE AND DISLOCATION

The most common fracture in childhood is that of the collarbone (clavicle). Suspect it after any fall when the child complains of pain in the shoulder below the neck. Take child to doctor for X-ray. Prevent dislocation of elbow (fairly common) by never picking child up by the arm or wrist, always by the underarm.

INSECT BITES

A damp cloth dipped in baking soda is soothing. Stinger may have to be removed. Doctor may prescribe antihistamine.

SWALLOWED OBJECTS

If blunt, these will usually be passed without difficulty. Regular diet should be followed. If sharp, as a pin or needle, bobby pin or open safety pin, observation by doctor will be necessary. Always close safety pins when you are changing diaper.

CHAPTER 17

How to Enjoy Traveling With Baby

WE HAVE FOLLOWED YOUR baby from birth to the age of a year-and-a-half. You have been able to watch him develop control over his body muscles and motions. Perhaps he is already gaining some control over his toilet functions. He hasn't developed the ability to "mind" you much yet, but he does want to please you. Control over his temper will be achieved through your patient guidance. From a small unresponsive being your baby has become a dynamo that reacts to everything.

Baby has now reached a stage where you can start venturing and adventuring forth more easily. Perhaps you have already taken several trips with baby. Babies go traveling a good deal and at a much younger age these days, for many reasons. Fathers and mothers change job locations or are moved about 5 times by their companies. Families of armed forces personnel sometimes follow in their frequent transfers. Vacation trips by car will frequently include baby (and several children) and can be delightful with enough advance planning.

SOME "DO NOT" TIPS FOR TRAVELING

Unless absolutely necessary, do not take a trip with a baby of only one or two months of age. You are both still making adjustments. Baby's schedule may not yet be regular enough to depend on. If you have a choice, flying is the easiest method because it is the quickest. Whatever the mode of travel, a car carrier is a must, even if you have to hold it on your lap on the plane.
It provides a comfortable place for baby. And you can pack many things into it, such as extra diapers and bottles. If you expect to travel by car to any great extent, you may have already invested in such a carrier and made use of it at home as baby's first crib.

And if you are traveling by car, under *no circumstances should you settle for anything less than a car carrier.* **Never place a car carrier in the front seat of a car if there is a passenger-side airbag**. Using a car bassinet, or holding baby in your arms is asking for trouble in case of a mishap. The first ride back from the hospital for your baby should be in an approved, backward facing car carrier and so should every ride thereafter until he is old enough to be strapped in, sitting forward like a "big person." The safest place for this car carrier or seat is in the center of the backseat anchored in place by the regular auto seat belt.

Infant car seats should be used until the child exceeds the weight limitations set by the seat's manufacturer. When this infant care seat is outgrown a toddler seat should be installed in the car ready for use.

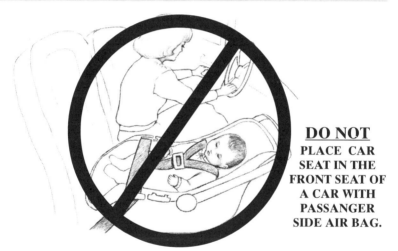

DO NOT PLACE CAR SEAT IN THE FRONT SEAT OF A CAR WITH PASSANGER SIDE AIR BAG.

The American Academy of Pediatrics endorses the following basic rules of car seat use:

- Always use a car seat
- Keep manufacturer's instructions with the car seat
- The rear seat is generally the safer position. There are only rare conditions where it is necessary for a child to be placed in the front seat. For example: A child with severe respiratory (breathing/lung) problems or seizures.

- The harness and/or shield holds the child in the car seat and the car's seat belt holds the seat in the car. Both must be attached tightly.
- The rear seat is the safest place for a child of any age to ride.

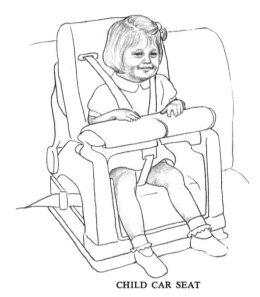

CHILD CAR SEAT

Toddler car seats are available for children weighing more than 17 pounds who are able to sit up by themselves. These seats face forward and are anchored by the car's lap belt which is either fastened around the front of the seat or threaded through the back of the car seat frame. The toddler is secured in the seat by seat harness. No child should ride in a car without being secured in an approved car seat until he is old enough and large enough to be secured in the standard auto seat belt.

Motor vehicle accidents cause the greatest number of injuries to children younger than 15 years of age: 4,000 deaths and 145,000 disabilities annually. Most states require a safe car carrier by law.

Do not travel with a sick baby or one who may become sick on the way because he has been exposed to a communicable disease.

Colds and other respiratory infections may become worse in the pressurized cabin of a plane. So if you can avoid it, do not fly when baby has a cold.

HOW TO HANDLE BABY'S FORMULA WHEN TRAVELING

If you are nursing the baby, accustom him to an occasional bottle of formula in case the breast milk supply fluctuates during the trip. Your doctor will advise you of the formula which is best for your baby.

The easiest formulas to take along on a trip would be the ready-to-use type, which requires no refrigeration or further sterilizing. If baby is not on such a formula, a few bottles of this may be tried out in advance.

Bottles of formula may be made up by terminal sterilization only for the first twenty-four hours of a trip. They should be chilled before starting out but will need no refrigeration en route.

If the baby is on whole milk, buy some cartons or bottles beforehand, though not too many if it's going to be a long trip, and ask to heat them up when you stop to eat. Or an electric bottle warmer may be plugged into a car cigarette lighter. The milk may not ned to be warmed if baby is used to having his bottle at room temperature. Baby could become accustomed to unheated milk in advance, too.

If you stop every night, you should stop fairly early as to be sure of getting accommodations and rest for all. Be sure to wash bottles and nipples thoroughly. If you chill the formula before starting out and can carry it in a cooler, you need not sterilize. Bottles of formula which have become very warm some time before using are best discarded. Milk is a culture medium that bacteria grow in under these circumstances. The same principles would apply to bottled and cartoned milk if you are carrying a supply of that. *Never use any raw, unpasteurized milk at any time for baby or anyone else.*

WHAT ABOUT WATER FOR BABY

Baby should have his own water supply lest variations in the quality and mineral content of the water en route upset his bowels. You can take boiled water in a boiled Mason jar with sealed lid. Or you can buy distilled water at a drug store in a half gallon jug. If you pour from it carefully and keep it capped, it should keep for several days or longer. A supply of paper cups will be used for water and juices. They can also be used for mixing cereal.

WHAT TO DO ABOUT DIAPERS

Diapers are no longer a problem. The disposable ones are a boon. These should be tried out ahead of time because occasionally a baby is chafed by them. Disposable diaper liners, although not so easy to find nowadays, are also good, especially if you can anticipate approximate timing of the baby's bowel movements.

HOW TO ENJOY TRAVELING WITH BABY

The cheapest method is to take baby's regular diapers in extra large supply. Many hotels and motels now have laundry rooms with coin operated washing machines for guests. And most cities have laundromats open till late in the evening.

Bring along a plentiful supply of plastic bags for the used diapers or a plastic pail with a tight fitting lid.

Scrupulous cleansing of baby's diaper areas, especially after bowel movements, is necessary when there are likely to be delays in changing. Cleansing tissues are helpful for this purpose. Take several boxes with you. Carrying a washcloth dampened with soap and water in a plastic bag is also useful. Washing may be preceded, as well as followed, by whatever lotion you are carrying. For long periods of wetness, such as at night, it is desirable to use some kind of ointment (not oil) to protect the diaper area. This could be plain vaseline, A and D or Diaparene ointment, or any your doctor has recommended previously.

CLOTHING

Clothing care is very simple and easy with modern drip dry fabrics. Keep a full day's supply as well as the diapers in a waterproof plastic shoulder bag so you won't have to scramble around in a suitcase. You could figure the approximate amount by a "dry run" at home. (Perhaps "wet run" would be a more apt description!) Always put in a few more of everything than you think you will need. The bag could also hold a plastic tablecloth and small cotton blanket for putting baby on, whether on car seat, on the ground or on the floor of a motel. Cleansing tissues should also be in the bag.

HOW TO KEEP BABY HAPPY

The child old enough to sit up will definitely want to do so. A good, sturdy toddler car carrier is absolutely essential. Such seats must be fastened to the rear seat using the vehicle lap belt to secure in place. Doors should always be locked. If baby clamors for your attention, do not be diverted while you are driving. Pull over to the side and stop. In fact, frequent rest periods for everyone to get "uncramped" are helpful. The smaller babies are soothed by the motion of the car and sleep blissfully in their carrier for many miles. But an older infant requires some distraction and play while traveling. No small child is interested for long in watching scenery go by. A favorite toy animal or doll, even blanket, must accompany him and be on hand, especially at nap and bedtime. For baby this small familiar token makes a "home away from home." A small toy suitcase can contain some well-loved picture books, crayon and paper, doll blanket and other doll "supplies." Perhaps some "surprise" may be tucked in. An old magazine to tear up makes a mess in the car but might keep a child busy for a long time.

Snacks should be carried in your bag, too, such as a teething biscuit, cracker, or arrowroot cooky. Small packages of cereal are also handy.

The baby might be entertained by your singing and talking to him and naming things along the way.

TOILET PROBLEMS

If you have room in the car, it may be a good idea to carry baby's toilet seat or a lightweight plastic potty chair that he is used to. If he is in the process of becoming toilet trained or has already achieved it, try to keep his usual toilet schedule. While training is often interrupted by a trip, the opposite may also happen. A child may actually become trained on the trip. Of course, this is due to the fact that he is developmentally ready, as happened in the case of Robert. His mother, a nurse, was worried for he was not yet trained at two years of age. When they went on vacation, he became "trained" very suddenly - in spite of the strange surroundings. His parents wondered if the fact that everybody was more relaxed about it had helped. Robert was very proud of his new achievement. Each time he "went" to the toilet he would say "Me do, Mommy." Indeed, it was his very own development that did it.

Babies do develop even while traveling. Enjoy your trip.

WHAT TO TELL BABYSITTER

1. All telephone numbers and addresses where you can be reached throughout the evening.

2. Your home telephone number and address and perhaps that of a neighbor who will be at home.

3. When you expect to return.

4. Your baby's doctor's name and telephone number.

5. Name and telephone number of nearest hospital.

6. Police and fire department telephone numbers. (Sheriff's number, if needed).

7. Poison Control Center telephone number.

8. Allergies or special medical condition your baby may have.

9. Specific instructions on bedtimes and foods to give baby in your absence.

10. All telephone messages.

MY POISON CONTROL GUIDE
(Post at every phone)

1. POISON CONTROL CENTER TELEPHONE NUMBER:_____

2. BABY'S DOCTOR'S NUMBER:_____

3. NEAREST HOSPITAL'S ADDRESS AND TELEPHONE NUMBER:

_____

4. Always save specimens of the poison taken for their examination.

5. Dilute the poison by giving the child liquids, unless you are advised otherwise. Any liquid will do which the child will accept. It is important to keep calm or the child will become panicky, too, and refuse to take anything.

6. If so advised, induce vomiting. This is best done with Syrup of Ipecac, but follow instructions on the bottle carefully. Putting your finger down the child's throat is dangerous and may not even work. Baking soda or salt does not always work, either.

7. Vomiting should start about fifteen minutes after administering the Syrup of Ipecac. When the child starts to gag, his head should be lowered over a basin so he will not choke.

8. EXCEPTIONS to the First Aid rule of making a child vomit the poison are few but important. In the case of corrosive poisons (drain cleaner, dishwasher detergents) or kerosene products (kerosene, lighter fluid, turpentine) and some others, vomiting may do more harm than good. This is why you MUST CALL YOUR DOCTOR AND POISON CONTROL CENTER FIRST.

BABY'S GROWTH HISTORY

Age	Height	Weight	Head Circumference
One month			
Three months			
Six months			
Nine months			
Twelve months			
Fifteen months			
Eighteen months			

INDEX

INDEX

INDEX

OTHER BOOKS IN THIS SERIES:

A MIRACLE IN THE MAKING

PREGNANCY
(Comprehensive edition)

A GUIDE TO PREGNANCY
& CHILDBIRTH
(Concise 5-COLOR edition) * & **

A DOCTOR DISCUSSES
NUTRITION DURING
PREGNANCY AND
BREASTFEEDING

BREASTFEEDING

A DOCTOR DISCUSSES YOUR
LIFE AFTER THE BABY IS BORN
The Postpartum Period

A DOCTOR DISCUSSES
THE CARE AND DEVELOPMENT
OF YOUR BABY

A DOCTOR TALKS TO
5-8-YEAR-OLDS

A DOCTOR TALKS TO
9-12-YEAR-OLDS

A DOCTOR DISCUSSES WHAT
TEENAGERS WANT TO KNOW *

A DOCTOR DISCUSSES
MENOPAUSE AND ESTROGENS

A DOCTOR DISCUSSES
HYPERTENSION

CREATIVE COOKING, Low-Sodium
(For Hypertensives and Their
Families)

A DOCTOR DISCUSSES
LEARNING TO LIVE WITH
STRESS, ANXIETY AND
NERVOUS TENSION

A DOCTOR DISCUSSES
HEADACHES

A DOCTOR DISCUSSES ARTHRITIS,
RHEUMATISM AND GOUT

A DOCTOR DISCUSSES DIABETES

CREATIVE COOKING, Sugar Free
(For Diabetics and Their Families)

A DOCTOR DISCUSSES ALLERGY:
FACT AND FICTION

A DOCTOR'S APPROACH TO
SENSIBLE DIETING AND
WEIGHT CONTROL

A DOCTOR DISCUSSES
CARE OF THE BACK

A DOCTOR DISCUSSES
CHOLESTEROL

* Available in Spanish
** Available in French

BUDLONG PRESS COMPANY • **Chicago, IL 60634-1403**